Living Pain *Free*

Healing Chronic Pain with Myofascial Release

A Self-Help Guide

Amanda Oswald

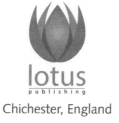

lotus
publishing

Chichester, England

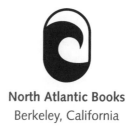

North Atlantic Books
Berkeley, California

First published in 2018 by
Lotus Publishing
Apple Tree Cottage, Inlands Road, Nutbourne, Chichester, PO18 8RJ and
North Atlantic Books
Berkeley, California

All Drawings Matt Lambert
Text Design Medlar Publishing Solutions Pvt Ltd., India
Cover Design Jasmine Hromjak
Printed and Bound in the UK by Short Run Press Limited

Living Pain Free: Healing Chronic Pain with Myofascial Release is sponsored and published by the Society for the Study of Native Arts and Sciences (dba North Atlantic Books), an educational nonprofit based in Berkeley, California, that collaborates with partners to develop cross-cultural perspectives, nurture holistic views of art, science, the humanities, and healing, and seed personal and global transformation by publishing work on the relationship of body, spirit, and nature.

North Atlantic Books' publications are available through most bookstores. For further information, visit our website at www.northatlanticbooks.com or call 800-733-3000.

British Library Cataloguing-in-Publication Data
A CIP record for this book is available from the British Library
ISBN 978 1 905367 81 8 (Lotus Publishing)
ISBN 978 1 62317 207 7 (North Atlantic Books)

Library of Congress Cataloging-in-Publication Data
Names: Oswald, Amanda, 1960- author.
Title: Living pain free : healing chronic pain with myofascial release / Amanda Oswald.
Description: Berkeley, California : North Atlantic Books, [2018]
Identifiers: LCCN 2017019417 (print) | LCCN 2017027741 (ebook) | ISBN 9781623172084 | ISBN 9781623172077 (trade paper)
Subjects: LCSH: Chronic pain--Treatment. | Massage therapy.
Classification: LCC RB127 (ebook) | LCC RB127 .O835 2018 (print) | DDC 616/.0472--dc23
LC record available at https://lccn.loc.gov/2017019417

Contents

CHAPTER 10
Typical Chronic Pain Conditions **129**

Acknowledgments

For Kahn

This book has been a long time in the making. Over many years I have subjected my nearest and dearest to my thoughts on fascia and chronic pain, so I would like to thank them for listening with varying degrees of patience, and for providing me with the necessary push in the right direction to actually gather those ideas into a book. I would also like to thank Jon and his team at Lotus Publishing for their patient guidance, and Emily and the team at North Atlantic Books for their unfailing enthusiasm for this project. Thanks also to Kieran and Lyz Igwe at Diligent Fitness, Leeds for the loan of themselves as photo models.

Foreword

Fascia has long been the forgotten tissue in the body, discarded by medical students as the 'white stuff' so they can get to the more interesting structures underneath such as muscles and bones. This disregard for fascia has arisen from a lack of understanding of the nature of the tissue, which often appears less uniform and more disorganised than other more easily identifiable structures such as muscles and organs.

Added to this, it is only recently that science has developed the tools with which to recognise and measure fascia. Even diagnostic tools such as X-Rays and MRI scans did not show this tissue adequately. However, more recent advances in ultrasound technology mean that it is now possible to identify the many differentiations in fascia in detail, from the tough ligaments and tendons, to the more fluid connective components.

Now scientists are beginning to be able to research what manual therapists have felt under their hands for centuries. And the field of fascia research is rapidly becoming an area of interest for many disparate disciplines, from scar treatment, surgery and rehabilitative medicine, to movement therapies and sports science.

The new terminology proposed for functional descriptions at the first Fascia Research Congress in 2007 defines fascia as all collagenous fibrous connective tissues that can be seen as elements of a body-wide tensional force transmission network.

The fascia is shaped and structured by the tensional forces placed upon it, which mean that it can be either tough and strong such as a ligament, or fluid and flowing such as loose membrane. Despite the names assigned to the different body structures by traditional anatomy, in the fascial world it is impossible to make clear distinctions or definitions between the fascia as it merges from muscle into sheath, into tendon and bone.

Force transmission too is no longer seen as something that happens between muscles as they contract and stretch to move bones. From a fascial perspective, a major portion of the muscular force is transmitted through the fascia surrounding these structures. This difference in perspective allows for the wider transmission of force throughout the body, instead of just a locally occurring event.

Fascia is also recognised as a tensegrity structure, a concept that served as a basic inspiration for the field of fascia research. Taken from arts and architecture, tensegrity structures are where the solid compressional elements are held in balance yet without touching each other, by the elastic tensional elements that are all connected to each other in a global tension-transmitting network.

In the body this translates into the bones being held in balance by the fascia, rather than the classical weight-bearing structure of the skeleton, as proposed in traditional anatomy.

There is much research interest into the load bearing implications of fascia when seen as a tensegrity structure. The fascial network adapts to the load bearing demands made on it, including the force of gravity which has evolved as humans have stood up and become bipeds. We now have specially adapted fascia on the outside of our thighs which enables us to stabilise our hips in walking, running and hopping. No other animal, not even our closest relative the chimpanzee, shows this kind of fascial feature. And even this feature adapts to use. For example, a runner or regular walker will develop stronger fascia on the outside of their thighs, compared with a horse rider whose inner thighs will become stronger with the demands of their sport, and compared with a paraplegic wheelchair user where the lack of use means any fascial strength disappears in their thighs.

These findings are of particular interest in the field of sports science and sports education, particularly with the rapidly advancing research into the ability of fascia to store and release kinetic energy. Put simply, correctly trained fascia has a greater ability to become more elastic, springy and resilient, leading to improved athletic performance and movement capability, while reducing the likelihood of injury.

What does all of this mean for the layperson, the general public?

Just as fascia can respond to sports training by adapting positively to sports-specific needs, so can it respond negatively to the ab-use of modern office life, a sedentary lifestyle and high stress.

Fascial thickening in the wrong areas can lead to restrictions which change posture and balance, reroute tensional forces and overload pain sensitive structures. It is these restrictions that can lead to many of the common chronic pain conditions that baffle the medical profession as they are unable to find an attributable structural cause. This is often because even thickened restricted fascia cannot be identified using common diagnostic tests such as MRI scans. And even if it was identified, many medical professionals have not yet been trained to understand the significance of the fascia they are identifying. The reason lies back in their student days when dissected fascia was stripped away as being medically insignificant.

As an understanding of the significance of fascia in body-wide health is now starting to ripple out through the sports world, it is important that this information is also shared with those people for whom the causes of their chronic pain have yet to be properly explained.

This book gives a clear and simple explanation of the fascial causes of chronic pain, and an introduction into ways in which you can help yourself out of chronic pain through your newfound fascial awareness. I am sure that every reader, whether coming from a lay person's perspective or from a health related professional background, will be able to get great value out of the following chapters; and to translate new inspiring insights into practical everyday applications for living a painfree and healthy lifestyle.

Robert Schleip
Director of the Fascia Group Project
Ulm University, Germany

Introduction

Millions of people suffer with chronic pain. For many of them, standard medical approaches are not working.

In the rush to promote big pharma and surgery, the holistic mind–body view of health has been abandoned, and the role of fascia, the main connective tissue in the body, has been neglected.

Fascia forms a three-dimensional web running through and around all other body structures including muscles, nerves, blood vessels, bones and organs. Fascia is the body's main source of structural support and plays an important part in communicating and maintaining chronic pain.

My journey into fascia started with my own chronic pain. I spent many years working long hours in stressful jobs, alternating long hours in the office with vigorous sports including rugby and long-distance running.

Like many people, I dismissed the warning aches and pains that came and went from time to time. And predictably I developed first RSI and then a prolapsed disc. Chronic pain set in and took over my life forcing me to stop working and abandon the leisure activities I loved. For several months I was confined to bed.

All I wanted was to be out of pain, so when surgery was offered, knowing nothing of the alternatives, said yes immediately. The miracle of disc surgery is that it can take the pain away immediately. However, what they don't tell you is that the scar tissue from the surgery can cause further complications. My pain changed and became less intense, but it didn't go completely. I could move again but was conscious of physical restrictions, and fearful of the pain returning.

In my efforts to heal myself completely, I re-trained and qualified first as a massage therapist then as a sports massage therapist. During my advanced massage studies, I heard about myofascial release and everything changed.

Myofascial release is a gentle non-invasive bodywork technique that works on the body's connective tissue – fascia – to release physical restrictions and pain patterns. Coming from an holistic tradition, it takes a mind–body approach, recognising that emotional experiences and trauma can play an important part in our experience of pain.

Once I discovered myofascial release, I wanted to learn everything I could about fascia. I trained with a wide range of fascia experts in the USA, UK, and Europe. I attended workshops and courses and fascia symposia, participated in fascial dissections, and read many, many fascia books. In this process I have benefited from the wisdom of others and made profound and life-changing connections of my own.

Perhaps the most exciting thing I have learned about fascia is how little we really know about it. Research into fascia has only become possible in the last 10 to 15 years as scientific instrumentation sensitive enough to detect and measure it has been developed. The things we are learning about the structure and properties of fascia are helping to explain how the body really works and offer a real life explanation for chronic pain. While the science catches up, myofascial release, and other fascial therapies, are working and providing effective treatment options for those for whom the standard medical approaches have not worked.

Over the past 10 years, in my clinic in Harley Street, London, I have had the privilege to work with many people experiencing a wide range of complex chronic pain conditions. Many have found their way to me after years of suffering, rounds of medical treatment, and having eventually been told they will just have to learn to live with their pain. Each and every one of them has taught me more about the relationship between fascia and chronic pain.

In return, I have treated them myofascially and explained to them what is going on in their bodies, why they have chronic pain, and how to take control of their own recovery so they can ensure their pain does not return.

This book is the result of my clinic work with clients. I've written it to share this knowledge and inspire as many people as possible to heal themselves fascially.

What this Book is About and Why I Wrote It

Fascia is the "Cinderella of the orthopaedic world" as it has been overlooked for so long, until now.

Robert Schleip, leading fascia researcher

My work as a myofascial release therapist

I am a myofascial release therapist, a complementary health practitioner. I qualified as a massage therapist and then as a sports massage therapist before doing many years of further training in advanced massage techniques and fascial anatomy.

For the last 10 years I have exclusively practiced myofascial release from my clinic in Harley Street, London, and traveled worldwide to study both the art of the technique and the growing body of scientific research that explains its success.

Myofascial release is a gentle hands-on technique that consistently gets results in "hard to treat" chronic pain conditions that other techniques literally cannot touch.

My clients and their chronic pain

There is a growing buzz around the phrase "myofascial release." This buzz is particularly strong in sports circles. People are starting to hear that elite athletes use myofascial release techniques as part of their training and rehabilitation programs.

For every sporty type who still believes the old adage "no pain no gain," there are tens, if not hundreds, of ordinary people who suffer from a wide range of chronic pain conditions and who would rather not experience any more pain, thank you very much. They are not necessarily athletes, they are not super-fit, and they have not developed their pain as a result of deliberately pushing their body to its limit. Their chronic pain has developed as a result of some combination of:

- accident and injury
- surgery and scar tissue
- the repetitive nature of their work or leisure activities (say, computers or gardening)
- their posture
- stress.

These people are my clients, and myofascial release is especially for them. They have all experienced chronic pain but range widely in age, from teenagers who suddenly develop debilitating headaches to octogenarians who can no longer walk properly after surgery. They can be office workers, musicians, yoga teachers, engineers, gardeners, bankers, full time mums. Some do regular sports and physical activities and some experience such bad pain that they can no longer do the things that they used to enjoy.

Medically they have been through the mill. They have seen their general practitioner, consultants, and specialists. They have had all manner of diagnostic tests and scans. They have been prescribed a cocktail of medication, some of which takes the edge off their pain but most of which gives them additional unwanted side effects. They have also tried a whole host of "standard" therapies, from physiotherapy to osteopathy, and often found them too painful to tolerate.

At some point, they have almost all been told that there is nothing more that can be done for them. Some have been told that it is all in their mind, which serves only to add guilt and shame on top of their pain.

My clients often tell me that they have come to me out of desperation because they have tried everything else. I am not offended or surprised by that – it is a comment on what has happened to them and the frustration they feel. They feel abandoned by the medical profession, confused, and exhausted by their pain.

My approach

Although many of the people I treat come to me with a medical diagnosis, I work with them holistically and in terms of their symptoms, not a label. This is because I have experienced many occasions when a particular diagnosis simply does not account for what my client is experiencing.

For example, I work with many people who have been given a diagnosis of fibromyalgia. This is a systemic condition, which means that it can affect the whole mind–body complex. There is a standard medical approach for the diagnosis of fibromyalgia and yet I have clients who have been diagnosed with fibromyalgia after spending 5 minutes with their general practitioner and others who have been diagnosed after a thorough consultation with a specialist. Some of those clients may have all the classic symptoms of the condition and are unable to work or live independently, while others hold down demanding jobs and regularly do long-distance runs feeling nothing more than the occasional niggling pain in their hips.

Self-help and self-empowerment

Knowledge is power, so I talk to my clients about their pain and offer them explanations from a fascial perspective. This new fascial self-knowledge, they tell me, makes sense to them and the simple fact of having it helps to ease both their anxiety and their pain.

When they want them (and sometimes when they do not), I give my clients suggestions for simple everyday fascial self-care techniques and exercises to help them take back control of their bodies and speed their recovery.

I personally have benefitted from hundreds of conversations with clients over the years. These have helped me to understand the information they have found most useful and the self-help help techniques they have found most powerful. I have set many of these out in this book so they can benefit others.

Who this book is for

This book is for all those people who are suffering with chronic pain conditions and who have been told that there is no cure. It is also for their families, partners, children, parents, friends, employers, and for anyone who wants to better understand a myofascial perspective on the causes of chronic pain and learn more effective ways to help themselves or their loved ones.

Chapter 2: What Everyone with Chronic Pain Has in Common
In Chapter 2, we look at the prevalence of chronic pain and at the causes of chronic pain. I outline what in my experience everyone with chronic pain has in common and the ways in which this affects their life.

Chapter 3: Bridging the Medical/Holistic Divide
In Chapter 3, I explain the medical approach to chronic pain and touch on the limits of the medical approach. I contrast the medical approach with the holistic approach.

Chapter 4: Why Holistic Approaches Are Now (Again) Being Taken Seriously
In Chapter 4, I explore the possibilities for a holistic approach to chronic pain and consider the science in more depth.

Chapter 5: What is Fascia?
In Chapter 5, we enter the fascinating world of fascia. We look at the anatomy of fascia and at how fascia functions in the body.

Chapter 6: Injury and Fascia
In Chapter 6, we consider how fascial injuries occur and how this affects fascia and general body function. We also look at how trigger points develop in fascia and muscle.

Chapter 7: How Chronic Pain Develops
In Chapter 7, we look at how the body experiences pain. We explore "normal" healthy pain and how this tips into chronic pain. And we consider the relationship between fascia and chronic pain.

Chapter 8: What is Myofascial Release?
In Chapter 8, we explain the hands-on therapy technique myofascial release and how this can be used for self-help.

Chapter 9: Help Yourself Out of Chronic Pain
In Chapter 9, we explore how a fascia-friendly perspective can inform powerful self-help techniques. We also introduce the principle of "slow fix."

Chapter 10: Typical Chronic Pain Conditions

In Chapter 10, we discuss some commonly diagnosed chronic pain conditions and contrast the medical approach with the fascial approach. We outline typical symptoms and offer a fascial perspective and an outline of fascial self-help activities and exercises.

Chapter 11: Fascial Activities, Stretches, and Exercises

In Chapter 11, we go into detail describing a range of self-help fascial activities, stretches, and exercises that can help to release your fascia and restore fascial health. We explain how to do each of the activities and stretches, and offer choices to suit your levels of pain and movement.

Chapter 12: Fascia in the Wider World

In Chapter 12, we offer some suggestions about ways to apply your new-found fascial knowledge to all areas of your life. We suggest ways to create a more fascia-friendly workplace, offer additional exercises, and encourage you to consider new forms of fascia-friendly movement.

Conclusion: Wrapping It All Up (in Fascia)

The conclusion offers a few final words of fascial encouragement for your journey out of chronic pain.

What Everyone with Chronic Pain Has in Common

Chronic pain is defined as pain that persists beyond the normal time of healing, or occurs in diseases in which healing does not take place. ... The Department of Health recognises chronic pain as a long-term condition in its own right, and as a component of other long-term diseases.

Chronic Pain Policy Coalition (CPPC)

This chapter includes:

- an introduction to chronic pain
- some statistics on how many people are affected by chronic pain
- an account of what everyone with chronic pain has in common.

Facts and figures about chronic pain

The "normal" time for healing is said by the Chronic Pain Policy Coalition (CPPC) to be up to 3 months from injury or other pain-causing event. Anyone still in pain after this time is said to have chronic pain.

The current estimate is that 28 million people in the UK live with chronic pain. In the USA that figure is 100 million people (Institute of Medicine of the National Academies). In other words, there are more people with chronic pain than diabetes, heart disease and cancer combined.

Of these people, more women than men suffer from chronic pain. The percentage of people with chronic pain increases with age. So, with an aging population both the number of people and the proportion of the population with chronic pain are set to rise.

In England alone, 3.5 million people said that their pain had kept them from their usual activities (home, leisure, and work) on at least 14 days in the last 3 months (CPPC). In other words, 3.5 million people are not able to work or get on with their lives because of chronic pain.

In 2008, the UK Chief Medical Officer's annual report highlighted pain as a major public health issue. It stated that 25% of chronic pain sufferers lose their jobs and 16% feel their pain is so bad they sometimes want to die (CPPC).

According to a recent National Institutes of Health statistics survey in the USA, the four most common types of chronic pain are:

Chronic pain	%age of respondents
Back pain	27%
Severe headache or migraine pain	15%
Neck pain	15%
Face ache or pain	4%

Apart from the pain itself, chronic conditions such as these are likely to affect general daily life. For example, American adults with low back pain are three times more likely than those without pain to be in only "poor" or "fair" general health, and more than four times more likely to experience serious psychological distress.

Direct physical injury, perhaps due to a car crash or sports accident, might be the most immediately recognizable cause of chronic pain, but the causes of chronic pain are complex. One major factor is the growing "sitting epidemic" in the western world. Sitting may sound like an enjoyable or fairly neutral activity, but it is affecting our health in many ways. Even those of us who do not work in an office sit too much. Typically, we sit to get to work (by car, train, or bus), we sit for most of our working day, we sit to get back home, and then, yes, we sit again to eat and to watch TV or use our computers in the evening.

This sitting epidemic has steadily grown over the last 60 years or so, starting with the introduction of labor-saving devices such as dishwashers and automatic washing machines, and continuing with the increase in car ownership, the invention of remote controls, increased use of computers, and so on. Even those of us who do not sit in an office for a living are likely to sit for around 10 hours a day; often virtually the only other thing we do is lie down to sleep.

We have reached a stage now where we hardly need to stand up at all, never mind move about. In fact, according to a survey by Public Health England (PHE), 43% of UK adults say they never exercise. And neither do we need to exert ourselves much, thanks to all the labor-saving gadgets and devices now in our homes.

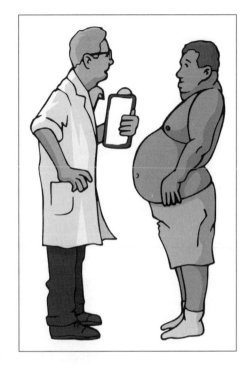

Figure 2.1: 43% of adults in the UK never take any exercise.

The problem of sitting is epidemic across the modernized western world. A global expert statement issued in 2015 by PHE and the campaign group Active Working states that 65–75% of an office worker's working day is spent sitting, over 50% of which is prolonged sustained sitting. In other words, office workers sit for many hours and they stay sitting in unnaturally fixed positions, rarely moving.

According to Active Working, there is a growing body of international scientific research that concludes that prolonged sitting is bad for your health, irrespective of the level of physical activity outside of work. Sitting can increase the risk of serious illnesses such as heart disease, diabetes, mental health problems, cancers, backaches, thrombosis, obesity, and muscle degeneration. All of these conditions or factors can lead to chronic pain.

The world depicted in the Pixar film *Wall-E* may not be all that far-fetched, where human skeletons have degenerated to the point that people have lost the ability to walk and have to be transported in hover-chairs.

Added to the sitting epidemic is the fact that many work tasks have become more and more specialized as employers seek out more cost-effective ways to get things done, without necessarily thinking about the human cost. Henry Ford invented the production line in 1913 as a way of streamlining car manufacture. Instead of one person, or a group of people, moving around a car to complete the build from start to finish, he realized that it was more time-efficient to move the cars along a conveyor and have workers stationed at specific points, each assigned to a single task that they did repetitively at speed as each car came past.

This approach certainly built Ford a lot of cars very economically, but his workers paid for it by contracting a form of repetitive strain injury (RSI) called vibration white finger. Vibration white finger was caused by repetitive use of the hands and arms to perform limited tasks that required force.

Likewise, office work has changed dramatically from the days of the typing pool. In the modern office the need to physically move anything more than fingers and hands is reducing.

Sedentary lifestyles and repetitive work are only part of the story. Although these factors may add to the persistence of chronic pain, they are not always the cause, and sometimes the cause can go unrecognized for many years.

As a myofascial therapist, I have spent the last 10 years working with people of all ages and from all walks of life, treating their chronic pain. Everyone I see is different and each person's chronic pain is as unique as they are. Everyone has a different history of how they have used their body, what work and exercise they have done, what injuries have befallen them, how their posture has adapted over time, and how they have coped with the stress of life and of pain.

How and why someone develops chronic pain varies from person to person, and many people continue to experience chronic pain despite visiting multiple medical specialists, taking medication, having surgery, and trying all sorts of therapies. The picture of chronic pain is a jigsaw of pieces.

However, over my 10 years treating many different people for chronic pain, I have noticed that they all have five experiences in common.

What everyone with chronic pain has in common

While the causes may differ, I have observed the following five factors that my clients with chronic pain have in common:

- Their pain is limiting their life.
- They have at least one medical diagnosis.
- They have had a lot of different treatments.
- They have been given a lot of medication.
- They have experienced trauma or are living with stress.

Their pain is limiting their life

Their pain has reached a stage at which it cannot be ignored. They are no longer able to work, exercise, do the things they enjoy, or even move comfortably without pain. As a result they no longer enjoy certain things as they once did and they avoid some activities.

The most typical symptoms people come to me with are:

- dull aches
- sharp electric pain
- constant nagging pain
- tingling
- numbness
- pins and needles
- inflammation
- loss of strength
- loss of movement
- stiffness
- fatigue
- insomnia
- anxiety.

Typically these symptoms move around and can vary in intensity, shifting and changing depending on the time of day, what someone is doing, how stressed they are, and how tired. Sometimes there just seems to be no logical reason for how the pain moves and other symptoms change.

Sometimes people have been living with these and other escalating symptoms for years and have accepted the limitations as inevitable. They are amazed when I explain what is happening to them and how it can be treated so they get back their pain-free physical movement and enjoyment of life.

Gillian, part 1

Gillian is a working mother in her late 30s. She has a busy lifestyle in and out of work. She has worked at a computer in an office for the past 10 years. A few years ago she was involved in a car crash and had a whiplash injury to her neck. Her neck was stiff for a while afterwards but this passed. More recently she has started to notice some pains in her hands. At first these just happened occasionally but now she finds that by the end of the day her hands are sore and feel swollen. At night she wakes and her hands feel numb and stiff. She is starting to drop things and become flustered. She has also developed a sharp pain behind her shoulder blade but does not think this is connected to her hands. Gillian is now starting to get quite anxious because she is secretly worried that there may be something sinister going on.

They have at least one medical diagnosis

Sometimes people have self-diagnosed following their own online research, but most often they have been given a diagnosis by at least one medical professional. Some of the most common diagnoses people come to see me with are:

- back pain
- bursitis
- chronic pelvic pain
- fibromyalgia
- frozen shoulder
- headaches and migraines
- myofascial pain syndrome
- plantar fasciitis
- repetitive strain injury
- runner's knee

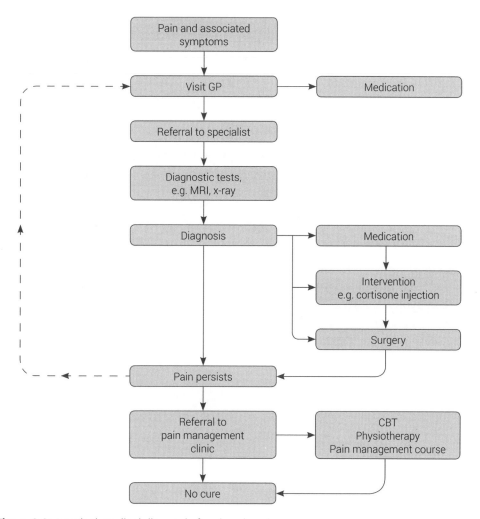

Figure 2.2: A typical medical diagnosis for chronic pain.

- tendonitis
- temporomandibular joint (TMJ) jaw pain
- trigger point pain

… the list goes on.

At this point I risk upsetting some people by saying that I do not set much store by diagnoses when it comes to chronic pain conditions, even when the diagnosis comes from a medical professional. There are two main issues with a diagnosis:

- There are massive inconsistencies, both in how people are diagnosed and in what they are diagnosed with.
- Although people may get a diagnosis, they often do not get practical help or support in how to alleviate symptoms or treat the diagnosed condition, which leads them to a sense of helplessness and despair, especially if the only option they are given is drugs or surgery.

The wide variety of symptoms that people experience and the way in which those symptoms shift around makes it difficult for someone to get an accurate diagnosis of their condition; and so can the way the medical system works.

Most people start their journey with a visit to their general practitioner (GP), who then sends them to a specialist. The type of specialist a patient is sent to depends on the predominant symptoms the patient has on the day they see their GP. If they have one set of symptoms they may be sent down one particular route but if their symptoms are different that day they may be sent down a totally different route. If those symptoms have changed again, or developed, by the time they actually get to see a specialist, this can affect both their diagnosis and their treatment plan.

Sometimes patients find themselves referred back to their GP to start again, or having inappropriate medical treatment out of a perceived need to "do something," even though the cause of their problem has not been fully understood or explained.

Perhaps this expectation that we must wait for and accept whatever medical diagnosis and treatment may be given is the reason doctors call us "patients"!

In many cases a diagnosis is no more than an educated medical guess, but a guess none the less, resulting from the natural human desire to help. Putting a label on a set of symptoms can help a medical professional produce a treatment plan, and it can help a patient to understand what is wrong with them. But does it?

I have seen countless examples of people being misdiagnosed, and having unnecessary surgery, medication, and treatment. In many cases, a diagnosis can have a negative psychological impact. A person becomes blighted by their medical label, spends endless hours trawling online forums, and is increasingly trapped in anxieties about their future prognosis, the lack of treatment options, and the lack of a cure for their diagnosed condition.

I have seen clients with the same symptoms and similar life circumstances receive completely different diagnoses, and I have seen clients who have been diagnosed as having one condition by specialist A and something entirely different by specialist B, because of the confines of those specialties.

As a complementary therapist I like to keep things simple – I do not diagnose, but rather I treat the symptoms as I find them, and I consider the whole person.

Gillian, part 2

After a really bad night's sleep, Gillian goes to see her GP. Based on the symptoms she describes, sore, stiff, and numb hands, Gillian's GP refers her to a rheumatologist, a specialist in conditions affecting the joints. In the meantime, the GP recommends she take ibuprofen and paracetamol (acetaminophen). When Gillian mentions that she has pain behind the shoulder blade as well, her GP dismisses that as being unrelated.

After several weeks, Gillian has an appointment with the rheumatologist who arranges for her to have an X-ray of her hands and a blood test for indicators of rheumatic disease. Gillian is told that she needs to wait several weeks for the test results. In the meantime, the specialist prescribes her some stronger anti-inflammatory medication and sends her home. At home, Gillian waits and researches her symptoms, which now include stomach pain and nausea, on the Internet.

Some weeks later she goes back to the rheumatologist, who tells her that the tests have come back clear and she does not have a rheumatic condition. Gillian is referred back to her GP with the suggestion that she see a neurologist.

After many anxious months, Gillian receives a diagnosis of carpal tunnel syndrome, a form of repetitive strain injury (RSI). At this point she is not sleeping well and has been prescribed an antidepressant to reduce her anxiety and help with sleep.

They have had a lot of different treatments

I have lost count of the number of people I have seen who have been sent from their GP to a medical specialist, to a therapist, and back again. Initially chronic pain sufferers will be treated using traditional medical approaches including medication, surgery, physiotherapy, and a talk therapy such as cognitive behavioral therapy (CBT).

Specialists they have seen may include neurologists, rheumatologists, orthopedic consultants, physiotherapists, occupational therapists. Then there may be further specialists involved, depending on where the patient feels their chronic pain; such as maxillofacial consultants for face and jaw pain, or gastrointestinal specialists for digestive pain.

Depending on their chronic pain condition and their consultant, people may have been given medication (see Table 2.1, below), pain relief procedures, surgery, or all three.

Pain relief procedures are generally injections directly into the painful area using drugs such as cortisone, Botox®, or anesthetics. The intention is to reduce the irritation in the area, and therefore the pain, and give the tissues time to repair and return to normal pain-free function. Often a patient needs to be sedated for the injection to be administered because the area being treated is so sensitive.

Depending on the pain condition, surgery may have been offered as a further option, and explained as a need to release pressure on a restricted area, such as the wrist in carpal tunnel surgery or joint decompression for frozen shoulder.

However, sometimes people are told there is nothing wrong with them, because diagnostic tests such as X-rays and magnetic resonance imaging (MRI) scans have come back as clear. They find themselves suspected of being a malingerer, or even told it is all in their mind, and are left with feelings of abandonment and hopelessness.

Some people may have been referred to National Health Service (NHS) or other pain management clinic, where they are told that there is nothing more that can be done and they must learn to live with their pain. These pain clinics are often run or managed by an anesthetist, which indicates the approach that is likely to be taken to chronic pain.

With no more help on offer from the medical services, people often conduct their own research and seek out other solutions. This might include therapies such as osteopathy, chiropractic, acupuncture, and massage. Often, the more therapists and specialists they see, and the more they read online, the more confusing and conflicting the advice becomes, to the point that they begin to believe that they really are untreatable.

Gillian, part 3

The neurologist who diagnosed Gillian with carpal tunnel syndrome recommends that she has a steroid injection into her wrists to reduce the inflammation which is normally associated with carpal tunnel syndrome. This reduces the symptoms in her hands for a few weeks but then they come back. She is then referred to a physiotherapist who recommends night splints for Gillian's wrists and gives her some exercises to strengthen her arm muscles. Gillian's symptoms worsen; one hand is now numb.

Gillian's neurologist explains that a ligament in her wrist is squeezing a nerve and causing her symptoms. They recommend that she has surgery to cut the ligament and relieve pressure on the nerve. Gillian takes time off work to go ahead with the surgery. Several weeks after the surgery, her scar has healed but her symptoms remain. At this point her specialist says there is nothing more that can be done and refers her to a pain management clinic.

Gillian starts to research alternative approaches.

They have been given a lot of medication

Before they come to see me, very typically people have started with a prescription from their GP for medication to help reduce their chronic pain symptoms. The problem here is that there is no drug specifically designed for chronic pain, and certainly nothing that can be given on a long-term basis without side effects. So most people are prescribed drugs that are actually meant for other conditions, but which are also known to have the effect of reducing anxiety, promoting sleep and relieving pain. The idea is to relax the painful areas and promote repair of irritated and sensitive tissues.

Table 2.1 lists some of the drugs typically used to treat chronic pain conditions, along with their common side effects.

Many of these common side effects are actually indistinguishable from the symptoms of the chronic pain condition they are prescribed to help. People on these drugs find it hard to tell whether their condition is getting better or worse, or whether any changes in their symptoms are caused by the drugs they are on.

Although I have talked about the common side effects that affect people who take these drugs (common meaning those side effects that affect one person in 10), others experience far more serious, even life-threatening, side effects.

It is common for people to be prescribed more than one of these drugs, and typically they will remain on them for several months, or even years. Often their prescribed dosage will be increased because the body becomes accustomed or resistant to medication after a period of time, at which point the drug stops being effective.

Table 2.1: Drugs typically used to treat chronic pain, and their common side effects

Drug	Common side effects
Amitriptyline (antidepressant)	Abdominal pains, chest pains, tingling, tiredness
Nortryptiline (antidepressant)	Anxiety, insomnia, nausea, constipation
Gabapentin (antiepileptic)	Abdominal pains, chest pains, tingling, tiredness
Diclofenac (nonsteroidal anti-inflammatory drug (NSAID))	Stomach pain, arm and leg pain, nausea, itching
Diazepam (for anxiety disorders)	Drowsiness, muscle weakness, loss of coordination
Tramadol (opioid pain reliever)	Headache, drowsiness, anxiety, tingling
Codeine (opioid painkiller)	Nausea, vomiting, dizziness, constipation
Morphine patches (opioid painkiller)	Drowsiness, lightheadedness, dizziness, sedation, shortness of breath, nausea, vomiting, sweating, constipation
Ibuprofen (NSAID)	Nausea, vomiting, diarrhea, indigestion, abdominal pain
Aspirin (NSAID)	Indigestion, nausea, vomiting
Paracetamol (acetaminophen) (painkiller)	Side effects are more rare but can include a rash and swelling, flushing, low blood pressure, fast heartbeat, blood disorders

I firmly believe that in future years, the over-prescribing of drugs to treat a chronic pain condition will be exposed as a dangerous risk to public health, as we now recognize the problem of routine prescription of antibiotics.

Gillian, part 4

At this point, Gillian has had steroid injections and surgery, and she is now on painkillers to take the edge off, anti-inflammatories to deal with a joint problem she does not have, antidepressants to alleviate the anxiety she is feeling, and now an antacid to calm the stomach problems caused by the other medication. She has noticed herself becoming irritable as well as feeling very tired and bloated.

They have experienced trauma or are living with stress

Talk about trauma and people tend to think of major life events such as a life-endangering accident or illness, loss of a loved one, or experiencing a war zone. All of these have a significant impact on the mind and body, and in the worst cases can trigger post-traumatic stress disorder (PTSD), in which the physical and psychological fallout from the event can negatively affect all areas of a person's life.

Short of these major traumatic events, there are many other relatively smaller traumas which can happen to people, such as minor surgery or accidents, or times of emotional stress. At the time, any of these events will temporarily increase the stress levels in the mind–body until they are resolved.

Everyday stress is also a natural part of life. It is the part of our unconscious behavior that keeps us safe from danger. Temporary stress, such as running to avoid a speeding car as you cross the road, can save your life and that is a good thing. Similarly, the temporary increase of stress on your body caused by a virus is also good, because it activates your immune system into fighting it off.

The problems start when people are subjected to repeated stress situations over which they feel they have little or no control. Much of modern life falls into this category, from job insecurity to your cancelled train to the endless menu choices of automated customer service "help-lines."

Over time these stressors can build up in your system to the point that your mind and body can no longer cope. After just 7 days of sustained stress your mind–body will go into a state of exhaustion where normal protective immune responses are no longer triggered and the body is vulnerable to disease and injury. PTSD is the most extreme reaction to this.

> **Gillian, part 5**
>
> Gillian is exhausted. She is not sleeping, she is in constant pain, and she has brain fog. She is finding it hard to do ordinary day-to-day tasks, and she has had to take time off work for the medical treatment and what has become a permanent cold. She is worried about losing her job. She is also having arguments at home, and her husband has suggested that it is all in her mind.

Many people who have chronic pain are in a similar state of exhaustion. Their chronic pain is a major stressor for the mind–body. The original injury or cause may, on the face of it, be healed but the physical pain has become chronically ingrained (in ways I will explain in Chapter 7) and the anxiety this causes feeds a vicious cycle of stress and pain. Breaking that pain cycle starts with recognizing and understanding what is happening.

While many people look for medical solutions, including drugs and surgery, in this book I explain why fascia, the main connective tissue in the body, is the holistic link to mind–body treatment of chronic pain.

Summary

In this chapter we have learned:

- Increasing numbers of people are affected by chronic pain conditions.
- Everyone with chronic pain has several things in common.
- Most turn to the medical profession for help before considering holistic therapies.

In the next chapter we will consider both the medical and holistic approaches to chronic pain.

Bridging the Medical/Holistic Divide

Mainstream medicine would be way different if they focused on prevention even half as much as they focused on intervention.

Anonymous

This chapter covers:

- why the medical profession separates the body from the mind
- the limits of this approach
- how a holistic approach to chronic pain offers an alternative.

Background to the current medical model

The current western medical approach has developed from theories that date from the earliest days of our scientific knowledge, a time when women wore whalebone corsets, men wore breeches, and illness and disease were widely regarded as a punishment from God. Two basic theories that are no longer generally considered to be true (ask any Buddhist philosopher or eastern healer) and current scientific research in many connected areas is proving conclusively that they are wrong. They hold that:

- body and mind are separate
- the body can be reduced to a linear, cause and effect model.

These theories, developed over 300 years ago, have their roots in the work of philosopher René Descartes and mathematician Sir Isaac Newton.

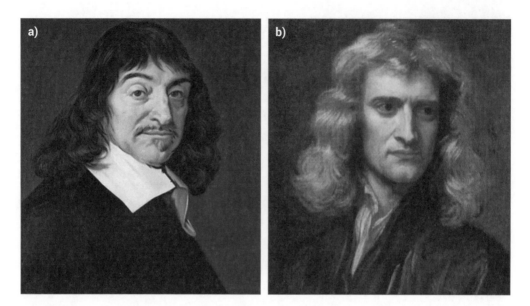

Figure 3.1: a) René Descartes, b) Sir Isaac Newton.

It was Descartes who first proposed the concept of mind–body dualism. He suggested that what until then had been regarded as whole and complete was, in his view, two separate entities – the mind and the body. This approach is known as the Cartesian approach (Renatus Cartesius being the Latin form of Descartes' name).

Descartes went on to say that the body was made of physical matter only and therefore could be studied scientifically, but since the mind was non-material or ephemeral it should be the realm of the Church.

At a time when science and the medical profession were challenging older forms of wisdom and the Christian Church was fighting to retain its influence, Descartes' view was accepted wholesale as the basis of a sort of ideological truce that suited everyone. Under the terms of this truce the Church claimed authority and control over the mind and the doctors took charge of the physical body. Both were careful not to stray into each other's territories, and so it remained, pretty well until Sigmund Freud came along and started looking into people's minds.

Meanwhile, Newton's ideas influenced how the body (and many other things) was studied. Newton created a branch of physics that looked for linear causes and effects and continually reduced what was being studied to ever-smaller units. The idea was to simplify everything to one single cause and effect that led to a single solution to an isolated physical problem.

The combination of these two ideas was how we lost our sense of the mind–body as a whole.

How the medical profession carves things up

The medical profession has continued to operate on the twin assumptions that the mind and body are separate and the body can effectively be reduced to a cause and effect model. This has resulted in:

- a disregard of those practitioners and therapists who have attempted to treat the mind and body as linked, and a lofty dismissal of patients with "psychosomatic" illnesses
- growing abstraction and medical specialization, splitting medical research and treatment into ever-smaller mechanical units, rather than seeing the bigger picture of mind–body health, and exploring the subtle energies that are contained within and which influence the body (and which are no less scientific, as we shall see)
- an emphasis on using physical means to treat bodily disease and illness; this has led to a focus on surgery and medication to treat body parts or symptoms, while the possibility of treating the whole person, including the social and environmental factors that influence them, has been neglected.

Medical research today looks more and more closely at ever smaller biological and chemical units in the body to locate the precise molecular causes of disease and to create pharmacological solutions in the form of medication (drugs).

As medicine and science have become increasingly specialized, so have the medical experts. We now have doctors and nurses who have detailed knowledge of their specialist areas, such as cardiologists, neurologists, rheumatologists, oncologists, endocrinologists, and so on. However, this specialist knowledge comes at the expense of an overall appreciation of patient health and the importance of holistic patient care.

While some medical attitudes have softened, and medicine has developed into mind-related areas such as psychiatry, psychology, psychotherapy, and so on, even here the approach has remained mechanical (electroconvulsive therapy) and chemical (drug) based.

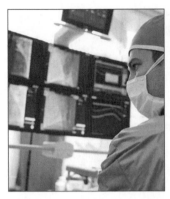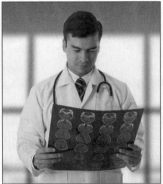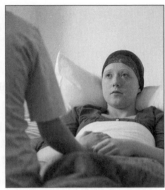

Figure 3.2: Medicine has become increasingly specialized, such as cardiology, neurology, and oncology.

In the west in the 21st century, we now find ourselves with a highly technical medical system that can treat diseases that would previously have killed people and can perform once impossible feats of surgery. However, despite these achievements, many patients who have received these specialist medical treatments have been left in chronic pain and been told there is no explanation and no cure.

This is because the old assumptions on which the medical system has been built have resulted in blind spots where the professions have neglected and dismissed those areas of inconvenient truth that do not fit their favored model. So while it is possible for a doctor to save your life by removing your ruptured appendix, medical professionals are also perfectly willing to dismiss your ongoing chronic pain afterwards as being "all in the mind" and/or nothing to do with their treatment.

The limits of current medical treatments

Our "modern" medical approach is still firmly rooted in the mind–body division inherited from Descartes and treatment is still based on Newton's linear cause and effect model. Treat disease A by blocking receptor B on cell C and the disease is stopped. Complex diseases, and relationships within the body, are simplified into models and treated as such.

Likewise, there is a focus on primary symptoms in one place and little regard for the possibility that symptoms elsewhere could be linked.

You might feel some aches and pains in your hand. You go to your GP who looks at your hand. If you describe your pain as severe enough, your GP will give you some medication to numb the pain.

If the pain persists, your GP may refer you to a specialist. This specialist could be a neurologist (specializing in the nervous system), a rheumatologist (specializing in joint disorders such as rheumatism), an orthopedic consultant (specializing in bones), or a hand specialist (a surgeon who specializes only in this area of the body).

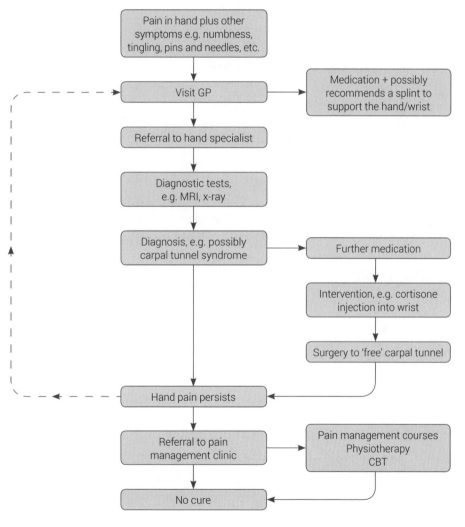

Figure 3.3: A typical path of medical diagnosis and treatment of hand pain.

The specialist will look at your hand and possibly run some diagnostic tests. They might order an X-ray, an MRI scan, a CT scan, or some blood tests. When those tests come back negative (as they frequently do) but your pain continues, the specialist may diagnose some vague kind of hand dysfunction.

Depending on their specialism, they are then likely to recommend surgery, more medication, or physiotherapy. If that does not work they will say there is nothing wrong with you or that there's nothing more they can do and you will have to learn to live with your (by now) chronic pain.

Throughout all of this they almost certainly did not look anywhere other than your hand for the physical cause of your symptoms. Nor did they consider your emotional wellbeing or mental health as a factor – either as a factor contributing to the original pain or as an understandable reaction to having undergone unsuccessful medical treatment and having persistent chronic pain. If the mind–body relationship was mentioned at all, it was most likely not until the drugs and surgery did not work and the doctor had no more answers.

For reasons we will discuss in Chapter 7, this specialist focus on where symptoms are felt and not where they originate does not work for chronic pain conditions, and nor does it reflect the complex reality of our bodies and our lives. A hand is not just a widget at the end of a lever that is an arm – a hand is a complex, living, organic structure made up of interconnecting systems and features and is just one part of a unique human being who lives a complex life full of feeling and emotions.

Offering alternatives to the medical approach

The current medical approach, with its mind–body division, has reached its high watermark. Science and society, however, continue to move ahead, leaving behind many of the attitudes and beliefs of the medical profession. Various social factors contribute to this:

- In the twenty-first century we are in an era of unprecedented strain on health services, commercialization of healthcare, and disillusionment with the limits of medical treatments. The current approach to chronic pain is a perfect example of this.
- Science has now disproved many of the assumptions on which medical research and medical practice have been based.

- A powerful combination of alternative research methods and widescale personal experience has proved that a more holistic approach to healthcare offers explanations for problems and alternative solutions.

Of course, if we are run over in the street we are still likely to need treatment in emergency and intensive care departments, but following that initial life-saving treatment we need to find non-medical ways to help ourselves through the trauma and to prevent or cure our chronic pain.

We can have the best of both worlds by considering when we need medical intervention and when holistic therapies and self-help offer better explanations and solutions.

Resistance to a holistic approach

Before the medical profession existed, people successfully treated a wide range of physical ailments and mental and emotional imbalances. They did so with a combination of hands-on treatments and traditional remedies. For these healers the mind–body connection was a given. These were the original holistic therapists in whose footsteps many current-day therapists have followed, continuing the tradition of treating the mind–body as a whole.

With the arrival of scientists such as Descartes and Newton came a new class and style of medical professional, keen to assert their superiority and to promote their two medical alternatives – drugs and surgery.

Resistance to holistic therapies has come almost exclusively from the medical professions and from those who profit from them, such as drug companies and private health insurers. This resistance works on many levels: dismissing holistic therapists as quacks, those who have experienced the benefits of holistic therapies as cranks, and those who wish to explore alternatives to medical treatments as misguided dupes who need to be protected.

However, there are growing numbers of people who have overcome this resistance. For many of them medical approaches simply have not worked, or have caused escalating problems, but holistic alternatives and complementary therapies have worked. And the growing interest in the use of holistic therapies to treat chronic pain does not just come from disillusionment with the shortcomings of the medical approach. Support for holistic therapies is gaining momentum due to an increasing amount of scientific and social evidence that supports their effectiveness.

But even now, each new piece of research is greeted by yet more resistance from medical professionals whose training has taught them that the mind and body are separate and who are absolutely unwilling to accept a holistic approach.

What this has to do with chronic pain

Chronic pain is an area in which there are no clear medical explanations:

- Medical approaches to chronic pain, such as drugs and surgery, do not work, and many people are left with chronic pain as a result of medical procedures.
- Chronic pain is costly both in financial terms and in terms of human suffering.
- A holistic, mind–body approach offers ways to understand chronic pain, alternative treatments, and self-help techniques.

Why Holistic Approaches Are Now (Again) Being Taken Seriously

Disturbances of the balanced state of health (together with psychiatric, social and economical problems) are now rarely viewed as illnesses, but are regulated to a position subordinate to illnesses, which can be objectively measured and put into scientific categories.

Alfred Pischinger, *The Extra-cellular Matrix*

In this chapter we will explore:

- challenges to the medical approach
- the scientific research that confirms the effect of the mind–body on health
- what this has to do with fascia and myofascial release.

The growing interest in holistic therapies to treat chronic pain does not just come from disillusionment with the shortcomings of medical treatment. It comes because millions of people worldwide have experienced the benefits of holistic therapies and every day new scientific breakthroughs are providing evidence of their effectiveness and explanations of how they work.

The holistic approach

We have seen in the previous chapter that modern medicine has a tendency to dissect the body into smaller and smaller distinct units in its attempts to isolate a single cause for every disease and illness.

By isolating individual elements in the body, medical researchers have created drugs that can target and affect those elements and which are now offered to tackle diseases previously thought untreatable. However, because no single part of the body is isolated from the rest of it, these drug treatments come with side effects that in many cases are at least as bad as the condition being treated. Even common over-the-counter painkillers, sold to us every day to treat headaches, can cause liver damage and stomach ulcers.

The increasing numbers of people living with chronic pain conditions that are resistant to treatment by medication, or who have woken up from surgery to find that their pain has simply moved elsewhere in their body, or now exists in a so-called "phantom limb," prove that the limits of this medical approach have been reached. It is becoming ever more apparent that treating the mind and the body separately is not the answer. And so interest in a holistic approach to human health is being re-kindled with the support of holistic therapists and their clients, and scientific researchers willing to follow the evidence and challenge the establishment.

The word "holistic" could accurately be written as "whole-istic." Holistic therapies are based on the fundamental belief that the human organism is a whole living system made of interrelated pieces. This approach is fundamentally different from the medical view in that:

- it recognizes the many levels on which elements within the body affect each other
- it regards the human organism as an open system that interacts with, and is affected by, the world around it.

From a holistic perspective, human health is a living, breathing jigsaw. Pieces in the jigsaw include what we eat, how we move (increasingly in this world *whether* we move), our social connections, our state of mind, the air we breathe, how much sun we get, and so on. Seeing the world like this opens up powerful possibilities for healing, and hopeful new avenues of scientific research.

New frontiers in scientific research

The medical approach to treating disease developed alongside early scientific methods. These methods largely relied on identifying and classifying objects and phenomena into ever smaller units, anything from butterflies (think of all those old wooden cabinets full of them) to bacteria. But as the results of research have accumulated and the limits of medical treatments and understanding have been reached, new forms of research have emerged.

The limits of drug research: the placebo and nocebo effects

For the whole of the 20th century and beyond, much medical research has been about trying to prove that drugs work, and that they work better than anything else.

Egged on by pharmaceutical companies in pursuit of massive profits, medical researchers have developed ever more abstract trials, determined to disprove the mind–body connection. The double-blind or triple-blind randomized controlled trial is now promoted as the gold standard for all research. These types of trial are expensive to run so only the largest pharmaceutical companies can afford them. Not only this, but the methods used in these trials do not always deliver the squeaky clean results the companies would have us believe. As a result, it remains unclear how, or whether, certain drugs work, and some drugs get "to market" despite evidence that taking nothing may be at least as effective.

In reality, in the wider research world, there are many forms of research evidence other than the randomized double- or triple-blind clinical trials that are accepted as providing robust scientific data. However, these methods are just as likely to prove the effectiveness of holistic therapies as they are to prove that drugs work. Drug companies therefore attempt to discredit these methods, while more and more researchers become disillusioned with this exclusionist and unscientific attitude and more convinced that a more inclusive, holistic approach to research and to human health is more appropriate.

The placebo effect
The placebo effect is basically the effect that the patient's belief has on that patient's experience of medical treatment. The word "placebo" comes from the Latin (*placebo*, meaning "I shall please").

The power of placebo was first noted by American surgeon Henry Beecher when he was working in a military field hospital in World War II. Beecher ran out of morphine when he was about to operate on a badly wounded soldier and was afraid that the shock of surgery performed without anesthetic would kill the patient. To his surprise, the theatre nurse calmly injected a syringe full of salt water into the solider as if she were injecting him with morphine. The soldier not only survived the operation but felt no pain during the operation or after it.

His wartime experiences led Beecher to direct his efforts towards minimizing the distorting influence the placebo effect could have on drug research. Beecher recognized that when a medical treatment was being tested on a patient, part of the apparent success of the treatment could come from the patient's hope or belief that the treatment would work. In 1955, Beecher published a paper that called for a new model of drug research in which one group of participants, chosen at random, would receive the real treatment and the other, a "control group," would receive a fake placebo treatment. Participants would not know which group they were in, so in theory the powerful placebo effect could not distort the results. And so the randomized controlled trial was born.

Initially researchers expected these controlled trials to clearly demonstrate the beneficial effects of the drugs being trialed. However, instead they demonstrated even more emphatically the power of the placebo. Because the members of the control group did not know they had been given the fake, they began to show improvements similar to those being given the drugs.

This was not welcome news for drug companies, so researchers cranked up their efforts to eliminate the placebo effect. It was suggested that because the researchers knew which participants were getting the real drug and which were getting the fake they were unconsciously treating people differently and therefore influencing the results. So the randomized double-blind trial was invented. In a randomized double-blind trial neither the participants nor the researchers know who is getting the active drug and who is getting the placebo.

However, even this level of trial still showed that people receiving the placebo could respond at least as positively as those receiving the real drug, and could get better.

The triple-blind randomized controlled trial was a further attempt to eliminate the placebo effect. In these trials even the analysts interpreting the results do not know who has received the real drug and who has not.

And yet the placebo effect continues to have a positive influence. There are now many trials in which the placebo has been shown to actually outperform the medication that is being trialed.

The positive effect of the placebo continues even when the participants in a trial know they are receiving a placebo. In 2010, in a Harvard University trial led by Ted Kaptchuk, 40 patients with irritable bowel syndrome (IBS) were given a bottle clearly labeled "placebo pills" and told that the pills contained an inert substance, like sugar pills, that had been shown in clinical trials to produce significant improvement in IBS symptoms through mind–body, self-healing processes. A second group of 40 IBS patients were given no treatment. After 3 weeks the group taking the placebos reported twice as much symptom relief as the no-treatment group – a difference comparable to the best IBS drugs on the market.

In another groundbreaking study in the late 1990s, by Jon Levine MS PhD at the University of California, dental patients who had just had their wisdom teeth removed were given placebos instead of pain medication. The patients felt no pain because, in response to the placebo, their bodies were producing their own endorphins, natural painkillers. To prove this, the researchers gave the patients a drug known to block the effect of endorphins. The patients' pain returned, proving that they had indeed been producing their own endorphins. This was a milestone in placebo research because it proved that the placebo effect is a mind–body response.

Something other than a drug treatment can create a healing effect in the body.

The nocebo effect

The flip side of the placebo effect is the "nocebo effect." When patients who have been taking placebos are told that the pill they have been taking is not actually effective, or that it is not a drug at all, they often become ill again. This is a demonstration of the nocebo effect.

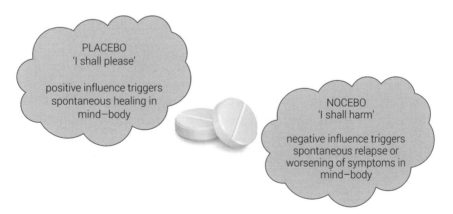

Figure 4.1: The placebo/nocebo effect.

The term "nocebo" was coined by researchers in the 1960s. It comes from the Latin for "I shall harm." A nocebo is an inert substance that causes a harmful effect simply because someone believes or expects it will harm them. The nocebo effect commonly occurs in drug trials and can occur even when a participant is not taking the real drug. It occurs in two subtly different ways:

- either, participants are told that they may experience side effects of some sort and then they do
- or, participants are specifically warned about the risk of a particular side effect, and they then report having experienced that side effect, even though they have not actually taken the drug.

The placebo and nocebo effects have produced such compelling evidence of the mind–body connection that many modern researchers have become less convinced about scientific methods that attempt to isolate individual factors and instead now study the science of belief.

The biological effects of thought on health

The placebo and nocebo effects mean that a person can alter and control their body simply by changing a single thought or belief. This is perhaps not surprising given what we have learned (above) about the power of the unconscious mind. This proof of the mind–body connection has in part led to the development of psychoneuroimmunology – the scientific study of the effect of thought and emotion on the immune system.

A wealth of research now exists to show that even our attitude affects our health and how long we live.

In 2002, the Mayo Clinic published a study that had followed 447 people for more than 30 years. It showed that optimists were physically and mentally healthier. Specifically, optimists had fewer problems with their daily activities. As a result of their physical health or emotional state, they experienced less pain, felt more energetic, had an easier time with social activities and felt happier, calmer, and more peaceful most of the time.

A previous Mayo Clinic study had followed 800 people for 30 years and showed that optimists actually live longer than pessimists.

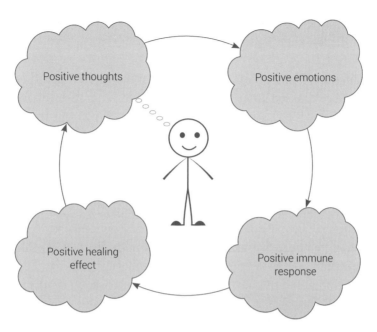

Figure 4.2: The power of thought = psychoneuroimmunology in action.

A Yale University study that followed 660 people aged 50+ for up to 23 years demonstrated that a positive attitude to aging sustained, on average, another 7 years of life. And that attitude had a stronger influence on longevity than blood pressure, cholesterol levels, smoking, body weight, or exercise.

With this knowledge it is easy to see how dismissal and hopelessness after failed medical treatment can affect a person's mental and physical health, and in turn their body's ability to heal itself.

It runs in my family – or does it? Genetics and epigenetics

The interest in the holistic approach to the mind–body is not news and there are increasing numbers of medical professionals researching outside the medical box. In his book *The Biology of Belief*, molecular biologist Bruce Lipton explains many of the flaws in current medical thinking in great detail. His work with stem cells led him to question role of genes and DNA in health and disease.

What is still an unproven theory about genes and DNA has become scientific dogma on which rests multi-millions of research pounds and dollars. The theory is that every one of us is born with a set of active genes that predetermines our susceptibility to particular physical and mental diseases. If our parents suffered from a genetic disease then we will too.

The gene theory leans heavily on Darwin's idea that the survival of a species depends on hereditary factors passed down from generation to generation. However, towards the end of his life Darwin had begun to doubt his own theory and to realize that environment also plays important role in survival.

Ignoring Darwin's change of mind, and in cause and effect mode, geneticists pursued the notion that specific individual genes control our physical, emotional, and behavioral health, determined before birth and unchangeable (talk about pessimistic). As a result, millions of people now live in fear that their genes will turn on them. Cancers, diabetes, heart disease, and many other serious diseases are said to be genetic and people feel helpless against a perceived inevitability that they too will inherit them. How many times have you heard people say sadly "it runs in our family"?

Not only is this belief likely to affect an individual's health in real ways, it is not true. The truth about the link between genes and disease has got lost in the media and funding hype.

While there is some evidence that certain faulty genes cause some rare diseases that affect less than 2% of the population, for example Huntington's chorea and cystic fibrosis, most of today's common diseases are not the result of a single faulty gene, but of complex interactions between multiple genes and environmental factors.

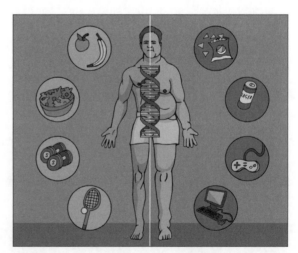

As researcher H. F. Nijhout summarized it in 1990, "a signal from its environment, not an emergent property of the gene itself, activates expression of that gene."

Welcome to the new scientific world of epigenetics, meaning "control above the genes." Epigenetics is the study of the

Figure 4.3: You are a product of your environment – most of today's common diseases are not the result of a single faulty gene, but of complex interactions between multiple genes and environmental factors.

influence on genetic expression of environmental factors such as nutrition, stress, and emotion.

Epigenetic studies have already shown that only 5% of cancer and cardiovascular patients can attribute their disease directly to heredity. A 2008 study by scientist and physician Dean Ornish revealed that just by changing diet and lifestyle for 90 days, prostate cancer patents switched the behavior of over 500 genes, many of the changes being associated with inhibiting tumor growth.

While it is important to choose our words carefully at this early stage of such research, it is clear that, far from being separate, there are deep biological and non-linear connections within the body and between the mind and the body that can be used positively for the benefit of our health. We will come back to these when we talk about fascia in Chapter 5.

Quantum physics

This may seem like an odd subject for a book about self-help for chronic pain, but quantum physics explains how holistic therapies work and why medical methods do not. As we shall see in Chapter 8, it also explains how myofascial release in particular works, so bear with me.

While western medical treatments remain stubbornly based on the ideas of the 17th-century mathematician and physicist Isaac Newton, physics itself has moved on.

In 1905, when Einstein came up with his equation $E = mc^2$, 20th-century physicists abandoned their belief in a universe made of matter in favor of the "discovery" that everything in the universe is made of energy. This is a discovery that, for millennia, has been a central truth of disciplines from martial arts to yoga and hands-on healing.

Quantum physicists now know that physical atoms constantly jiggle, spin, and vibrate. In doing so they attract those other atoms that jiggle, spin, and vibrate at the same rate or frequency. Atoms, being made of energy, have no physical structure themselves, but when they come together at the same frequency they create the illusion of solidity.

In other words, the world we live in is constantly forming and re-forming and we are all part of one indivisible dynamic whole in which energy and physical matter are so deeply connected it is impossible to consider them as independent elements.

This quantum universe in which we live is a truly holistic universe. In this universe it is easy to understand the mind–body connection, the power of mind over matter, and the healing power that can come from physical touch and emotional support. But this is only one way in which quantum physics is relevant to holistic therapies.

Earlier in this chapter we discussed the medical research world's attempts to use randomized double-blind and triple-blind tests to isolate a single factor or drug and prove that it works. Quantum physics has now shown that the interconnected universe does not work like that. More than that, it has also shown why those test methods cannot ever work to explain the effectiveness of holistic therapies. The reason is simple and it is one we can all relate to: atoms change their behavior when they are being observed.

This simple truth about atoms has two profound implications for methods of healing and for self-help:

- despite masses of evidence that holistic therapies work, it explains why it is so hard to "prove" they do in medical terms.
- it also means that the very act of paying attention to something, for example a painful shoulder, can change the way in which the cells and tissues in the shoulder behave and this offers possibilities for healing.

Possibilities for the holistic treatment of chronic pain

Research into alternative therapeutic approaches is not new or "wacky." In fact, researchers in leading university laboratories have been looking at holistic and energetic approaches to healing since the 1930s.

A fascinating example is the pioneering work of Harold Saxton Burr, Professor of Anatomy at Yale for over 40 years. At Yale, Burr began a series of important and controversial studies of the role of electricity in disease. Over time he published more than 90 scientific papers on the subject and was involved in another 100 or so. Burr discovered that all living things, plant, animal, and human, had an electromagnetic "field of life" that could be measured with a basic voltmeter. He believed that this field of life was a blueprint that created form and shape and being. It was what made a tree a tree and made a human, human. Burr believed that by studying this energy, it was possible to diagnose the physical and psychological state of an individual. From this he concluded that it is possible to use natural "healing energy" to correct any imbalance or disease in the field of life and restore health.

Burr was way ahead of his time and he was very aware of this. In the period between 1916 and 1956, when he was publishing his research, the medical world was focused on mechanical and pharmaceutical advances and his work was neglected and ridiculed. But modern research by energy researcher Dr James Oschman and others has now confirmed Burr's findings. Every event in the body, either normal or pathological, produces electrical changes and alterations of the magnetic fields around the body.

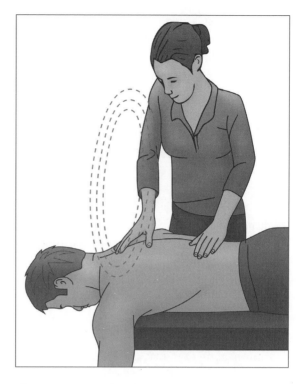

Figure 4.4: Natural healing energy from the therapist's hands connects and intermingles with that of the client, helping to correct imbalances and restore health.

One of Burr's most controversial areas of research was the use of energy fields for early detection of cancer, before tumors developed. Modern research now repeatedly shows that the presence of viruses, bacterial infections, cancerous tumors, and diseases such as AIDS can all be measured as disturbances in the energetic fields of the body.

The study of bioenergy fields has gone from scientific "nonsense" in the time of Burr, to an important and expanding subject of biomedical research. But it will be a while before the research is incorporated into medical training and available to the public. In the meantime, the research confirms much anecdotal evidence from individuals and holistic therapists.

William Redpath, a therapist and sufferer of stored trauma caused by abuse, went through a profound process of release and resolution and now works to heal others. He believes that the processes that enable healing to occur in both hands-on and hands-off therapies are electromagnetic and that quantum physics explains why they cannot yet be fully observed.

They can be explained by something called "microgenesis," which describes how consciousness moves in electromagnetic brain waves (each lasting about one-tenth of a second) that flow through and out of the body. The repeated flow of brain waves, each overwriting the last, is what creates consciousness.

Microgenesis is demonstrated by those moments when time seems to slow down. These moments are frequently reported by those who have gone through a serious accident or life-threatening situation. They are thought to be the result of the brain producing additional consciousness units to enable the body to take rapid life-saving action.

Migrogenesis is important for holistic hands-on therapies because it helps account for the significant moments of realization or insight and resolution that can occur in therapeutic sessions. One theory is that these moments happen when an electromagnetic wave of consciousness meets a stored trauma within the body and resolves it.

In terms of massage this might be no more than soothing away the stresses of the day, but healing of injury, chronic pain, and other trauma is also possible.

What this has to do with fascia and myofascial release

As we will see in the next chapter, fascia is the main connective tissue in the body, physically connecting muscle with bone and everything with everything else. Fascia is also capable of creating, storing, and conducting electromagnetic energy at speeds faster than the nervous system. Myofascial release is a hands-on bodywork technique that works on fascia with a positive understanding of the energies and emotions that shape physical health.

What is Fascia?

The soul of man with all the streams of pure living water seems to dwell in the fascia of his body. When you deal with the fascia, you deal and do business with the branch offices of the brain.

Andrew Taylor Still MD, 1899

Fascia is the soft tissue component of the connective tissue system that permeates the human body forming a whole-body continuous three-dimensional matrix of structural support. It interpenetrates and surrounds all organs, muscles, bones and nerve fibers, creating a unique environment for body systems functioning.

Fascia Research Conference, Harvard, 2007

In this chapter we will:

- unlearn some of what we thought we knew about anatomy
- discover something about the structure and properties of fascia
- begin our exploration of fascial ways to treat injury, disease, and chronic pain conditions.

Introduction to fascia

Fascia has two main roles in the body:

- physical support
- communication.

Fascia is the main connective tissue in the body, connecting everything to everything else. The ligaments that hold our joints together and the tendons that connect the muscles to the bones are all made of fascia. But it does not stop there. As we examine the body more closely we find that fascia wraps around and runs through every one of its structures, protecting them and giving them shape. Fascia encases and runs through organs such as our heart, blood vessels, nerves, and the muscles that make our limbs work. Going deeper, fascia holds together every cell and every fiber that makes up those organs, connecting each of them to its neighbors and, through a vast network, connecting everything with everything else. Your knee bone is indeed connected to your thigh bone, but not in the way you think.

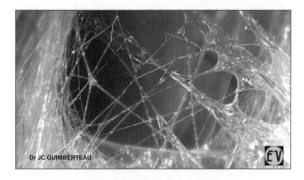

Figure 5.1: An image of fascia in the living body which depicts it as a fully interconnected three-dimensional network. *Photograph courtesy of Dr. J. C. Guimberteau.*

If you have ever prepared a chicken breast for dinner you will have encountered fascia – it is the almost invisible filmy-white surface membrane that gets snagged and wrinkled as you handle the meat. (Those who do not eat meat might prefer to think of the layers of pith that wrap around an orange, just under its skin, and the thinner seams that run around and through each segment and cell.)

As well as having a role in physical balance, this connective network of fascia within the body is a communication system that works quicker than your nervous system.

To really appreciate the role of fascia within our bodies we must first unlearn some traditional anatomy.

Unlearning traditional anatomy

Traditional anatomy is taught to medical and nursing students. Medical students spend many hours in the dissecting lab looking in detail at the structures of the body. To do so, they are told to strip away the "white stuff" so that they can get to the more important structures beneath, such as muscles, bones, and nerves.

This "white stuff" that the students discard in the dissection lab is fascia. Although fascia is the most widespread tissue the body, it does not fit into the traditional categories for study, so the role and importance of fascia has not been widely recognized or taught.

Traditional anatomy divides the body into separate cells, tissues, and systems, and the medical profession has developed into separate specialties that match these systems. In doing so it has moved away from regarding the mind–body as an interconnected whole.

Cells are the smallest structures in the body capable of independent life and of reproducing themselves. There are about 50 trillion cells in the body. Each cell contains its own units for energy production, storage, and waste disposal, and factories producing new substances. Cells live in a watery environment and depend on the fluid surrounding them to deliver nutrients, remove waste products, and communicate messages and instructions.

An individual cell is held together by the walls that surround it and which contain its internal structures. Cells are also bound together, like with like, into body tissues.

These body tissues have been categorized based on their function and consistency. And these different tissues are said to combine into body systems, for example the muscular system and the nervous system.

While the categorization of body tissues and the division of the body into separate systems may be familiar to us, and is generally accepted as fact, it is just one way of breaking down a complex structure we do not quite understand into smaller units that are easier to study. It is a way of ordering our thoughts, to try to make sense of what might otherwise appear messy and chaotic, and to explain how the body works.

The two major downsides of this approach are that:

- The divisions we have created are false and do not actually exist. The biggest of these is the mind–body division.
- Things may actually work differently from how we imagine and do not work according to the explanations that arise from these false divisions. This is particularly relevant for the study of chronic pain.

Dividing the body along the lines of traditional anatomy forces students of traditional anatomy to disregard or downplay certain lived experiences that cannot be explained in terms of traditional anatomy. This means that the medical profession may sometimes be looking in the wrong direction, or looking at things in the wrong way.

Traditional anatomical tissues and body systems

Classifying the body into separate tissues and systems and treating them in separate specialties is problematic. Table 5.1 shows a breakdown of major body systems and the tissues and organs within those systems.

From a quick look at this table it is possible to see that, although they might be presented as separate, these systems and their functions are all interrelated. For example, the digestive system provides the energy for the muscular system, which in turn moves the skeletal system. Which muscles move which bones and in what direction is determined by signals from the nervous system, which also has a role in controlling the digestive system. And so it goes on.

Taking it back a level to the body tissues that make up the systems, these are not clear-cut. As we have already seen, tissues are classified according to both function and consistency. Connective tissue appears in all of the categories, and whatever its consistency, all connective tissue, whether it is blood or bone, contains fascia.

If we take it back another level, even our cells do not necessarily belong to one category of cell or another; most cells start life as multi-purpose, with the potential to be any sort of cell, and only become shaped to a particular purpose if that is what our body needs at the time.

Despite all of this overlap and ambiguity, the medical professions have organized themselves into specialties that closely mirror the anatomical divisions. In doing so they have limited their ability to see connections or to treat the messy reality of certain conditions that blur the boundaries.

We have cardiologists, gastrointestinal specialists, orthopedic consultants, neurologists, endocrinologists, and so on. Each focuses on their specialism and each offers medical solutions that fit the Newtonian cause and effect model: medication, surgery, or both.

Table 5.1: The traditional medical approach to how anatomy is taught as independent tissues and body systems

System	Tissues and organs
Cardiovascular system	Heart, blood vessels, and blood – responsible for delivering oxygen and nutrients to every cell in the body and removing waste products
Digestive system	A series of tubes from mouth to rectum and including your stomach, pancreas, liver and gall bladder; it is responsible for breaking down the food and drink we ingest so that our cells can use them. The liver is almost a system in itself, performing over 500 essential functions
Endocrine system	Sends and receives messages in the form of hormones, tiny chemicals that create massive changes in the body
Immune system	Glands that protect us from disease, bacteria, and viruses – the thyroid, tonsils, adenoids, spleen, appendix – and the lymph nodes and glands
Integumentary system	Skin, hair, and nails – our outermost protection system
Lymphatic system	Lymph fluid and vessels, lymph nodes and glands which drain excess fluid from our tissues back into our blood and help to protect us as part of the immune system
Muscular system	Formed of our cardiac, smooth, and skeletal muscles
Nervous system	Collects signals from nerve endings in tissues in all parts of the body and sends these to the brain to be interpreted. Transmits instructions back from the brain to the rest of the body
Reproductive system	Uterus and ovaries in women; penis, testes and prostate in men
Respiratory system	Lungs and associated muscles – responsible for oxygen intake and carbon dioxide removal
Skeletal system	Bones and joints
Urinary system	Kidneys, bladder and associated "tubes" which process, filter, and dispose of waste products from the body

Sometimes, this focus can be a good thing. Modern surgical techniques and medication have saved countless lives. Surgery to cut out cancer or a perforated bowel can be a lifesaver, and many horrible diseases have been eradicated or become increasingly rare due to pharmaceutical breakthroughs. However, this focus can also have unintended consequences. For example, life-saving surgery can be followed by the development of chronic pain, often years later, in another and seemingly unconnected part of the body.

Similarly, if you talk to a medical specialist about the pain in your hand and mention your headaches, they will dismiss these as being totally unconnected. Likewise, the gastric specialist will not link the pains in your knees to your abdominal bloating and IBS. But these conditions and symptoms are all interlinked and can develop as a result of imbalance between these parts.

Because the divisions on which we base medical treatments simply do not exist in the way we imagine, and because the body is actually an interconnected whole, when we intervene in one area we change the whole balance throughout the body. If this intervention willfully ignores certain things that simply do not fit with our way of looking at things, like the medical students scraping away fascia to get to the more "interesting" bits, then we cannot be surprised when puzzling problems arise to which the medical approach has no answers.

Complex chronic conditions, such as fibromyalgia and ME, and chronic pain are all examples of messy human experience that puzzle the medical profession, and which many of them are tempted to dismiss. But fascial therapists have found answers, based on an alternative and holistic view of the body. Which brings us to fascial anatomy.

Fascial anatomy

Fascia is not a new thing. The quotation at the beginning of this chapter comes from Andrew Taylor Still and was written in 1899. Andrew Taylor Still is known as the "father of osteopathy." He recognized the importance of fascia both in its relationship with muscles and bones and on a deeper and more profound level as part of a communication system connected with the brain. In both of these senses fascia can be regarded as the "connecting connective tissue," connecting everything with everything else.

At around the same time, D. D. Palmer, the founder of chiropractic, wrote of a "controlling intelligence ... able to transmit mental impulses to all parts of the body, free and unobstructed." He was referring to a function of fascia.

Despite their early holistic and fascial roots, both osteopathy and chiropractic have taken a different (more linear) path and now many osteopaths and chiropractors work without an understanding of fascia. This is disappointing but unsurprising as throughout the 20th century, as osteopathy and chiropractic became recognized medical disciplines, the study of fascia fell out of medical and scientific fashion.

Despite greater interest in previous centuries, the current edition of the standard medical text book *Gray's Anatomy* devotes a mere page and a half out of over 1,500 pages to fascia. According to *Gray's*, fascia may be useful, or "functionally significant," in areas such as arteries, and helpful as a connective tissue, but otherwise it is a packing material.

Apart from medical skepticism about holistic connections, the main reason the study of fascia has fallen out of fashion is that we have only recently developed instrumentation to effectively and accurately analyze and measure fascial behavior. Now, in the 21st century, in university research laboratories across the world, new techniques in scientific research are starting to show the significance of fascia in the mind–body whole.

The fascial web

Fascial anatomy takes a completely different perspective from traditional anatomy. Rather than dividing the body into ever smaller functional units or systems, fascial anatomy recognizes that fascia is found everywhere, at every level in the body. Fascia forms the sheaths that encase muscles and tendons,

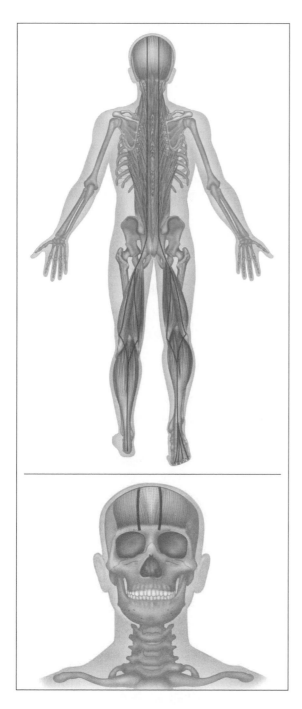

Figure 5.2: These images of fascial lines in the body demonstrate how a restriction in one area can create pain in another as the tensional forces travel along these lines.

it gives strength to ligaments and bones and fluidity to blood and body fluids, it surrounds organs, blood vessels, and nerves and fills body cavities, providing protection and support. Fascia connects the skin to deeper organs and structures; it even forms the internal structures of cells themselves. In doing all of these things fascia forms a three-dimensional web throughout our bodies.

In its normal state, fascia is fluid, containing a high proportion of water, consistent with the 70% water content of our bodies. This high fluid content enables fascia to move freely as we move and to constantly shift shape and adapt its complex three-dimensional network to every demand we make of it. Damage fascia, however, and this creates a pull or snag in the web, similar to a snag in a jumper or a pair of tights that bunches up around a hole and begins to pull on neighboring areas.

Certainly fascia merges and blends with every other structure in the body in a way that makes it impossible to separate one from the other in either a living or a dead body without a very sharp scalpel and a lot of precision and force. Nevertheless, some researchers have been trying and have succeeded.

Tom Myers is an early new wave fascia researcher and therapist who has contributed much to the understanding of the how fascia connects within and across the body.

Through extensive cadaver dissection focusing on fascia Tom Myers has developed the concept of "anatomy trains." Instead of the traditional view of the body as a series of separate units, he has teased out and traced lines of fascia that connect the body's moving parts. His research reveals that in reality, you cannot separate muscles from tendons or tendons from bones, or even one muscle from another muscle. All are part of one continuous fascial network.

Within this network, Myers has traced a series of lines, or meridians, each of which describes a very precise line of fascial tension or pull through the body. These meridians run superficially (that is, near the surface of the skin) or deep (affecting organs and deeper structures); they run up the back, front, and sides; and they even run in spiral lines round the body like a helter-skelter.

By tracing these meridians, it becomes possible to see how a minor accident such as spraining your right ankle can have a long-term effect on your left shoulder as the strain of your injury is transmitted along the fascial meridian line that spirals from one to the other. Or how those headaches you keep getting might be caused by a torque or twist in your spine that runs from your pelvis up into your neck. It also explains why, in my experience as a fascial therapist, it is possible to get rid of a client's persistent headaches by correcting an imbalance in their pelvic bones that has been causing distorted tension in the fascial network.

Another leading fascia researcher and therapist, Robert Schleip, has taken this idea of functional forces further to suggest that muscles are not the all-important movers and shakers we might once have thought. Schleip has stated that muscles are simply the housing for "motor units" that create the energy that powers "a complex network of fascial sheets, bags and strings that convert [it] into the final body movement." In Schleip's view it is the fascia that creates and directs movement, not the muscles.

From a similar fascial perspective, tutor and therapist James Earls has noted that "we use the whole body to walk: the pelvis and legs are assisted by the trunk and the arms. The whole body helps balance and movement by increasing and decreasing the forces moving through the soft tissue."

This idea of fascia as transmitting the overall connecting force in the body is a research topic being studied by other modern fascia scientists. At the forefront of these is the Stecco family. Father, Luigi Stecco, a physiotherapist, developed a practical and effective fascial treatment technique based on what he could feel when working with the body. His children Carla and Antonio, both medical doctors, are working now to prove this scientifically. In fact, much of the research currently being conducted on fascia is proving what therapists have felt under their hands for centuries.

Through painstaking research over many months, which she described as being "locked away" in a cadaver lab, Carla Stecco has separated out the layers of fascia to explain how even the most superficial touch of the skin can have a profound effect deep into the body.

What Carla Stecco has shown is that underneath the surface of the skin there are tiny vertical fascial threads that communicate

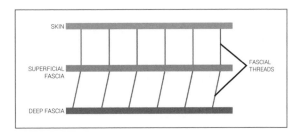

Figure 5.3: Fascial threads attached to the underside of the skin communicate directly to a layer of superficial fascia a few millimeters below. Further fascial threads connect from the superficial fascia down to the deep fascia. The vertical threads conduct touch very directly to the superficial fascia, while the diagonal threads exert a more subtle pressure that creates movement deep within the body.

directly from the skin to a layer of superficial fascia a few millimeters below. From the superficial fascia there are then millions and millions more fascial threads arranged diagonally in layers leading down to the deep fascia surrounding and supporting our internal organs and other structures. The vertical threads conduct touch very directly to the superficial fascia while the diagonal threads exert a more subtle pressure that creates movement deep within the body.

And it does not stop there. The Steccos have identified the relationship between fascia and other structures within the body. Throughout the body, fascia has been shown to adapt and split in many places to allow structures such as fat cells, muscle tissue, blood and lymph vessels, and nerves to pass through or be accommodated.

This close connection with other body structures is what has led some researchers to suggest that fascia is not just a connective tissue but is actually the tissue from which all other tissues originate.

What fascia is made of

The two main components of fascia are:

- protein
- water.

Protein

Proteins are the building blocks of the body. Fascia is made of two main proteins:

- collagen for strength
- elastin for flexibility.

These two proteins are what give fascia its physical form, and that physical form exists throughout the body in a web that runs around and through our cells, nerves, organs, bones, muscles, and skin, connecting everything with everything else.

Fascia also contains a finer mesh of smaller proteins that bind together and hold water within the fascia.

The proteins from which fascia is built are created by genes and, as we have seen in Chapter 4, the production of proteins can be affected by changes in behavior and thought.

Water

Fascia is the main connective tissue in the human body and the human body is 70% water on average, so it is not surprising that the second main component of fascia is water.

The relationship between water and fascia works in two ways. First, water gives fascia the fluidity it needs for movement. Second, the water within fascia holds and releases energy.

Seen under a microscope, fascia looks very beautiful – like a spider's web with dewdrops caught between the strands of web.

This fascial web works in three dimensions capable of infinite movement in many directions at once. As the fibers within the web move they cross and re-cross each other, dividing and re-joining in an elegant dance, while the web constantly forms and re-forms, adjusting to the stresses and strains placed on it.

To learn more about what fascia looks like, take a look a one of the videos produced by Jean-Claude Guimberteau. Guimberteau is a French surgeon who used a tiny camera inserted under the skin to record the movement and beauty of living fascia. His videos are works of art, and clips of them can be seen on YouTube.

As well as superficial fascia immediately under the skin, the body also contains deep fascia on a larger scale. Consider the array of internal organs we all (mostly) have packed tightly into our abdominal and pelvic cavities: the liver, stomach, kidneys, spleen, bladder, and uterus or prostate, not to mention the 9 meters of tubing that is the digestive tract. Each of these organs needs to maintain its own space and yet must be able to respond to our movements. Even a simple action such as bending over to tie our shoelaces requires all of these organs to shift and slide freely to maintain a harmonious environment. It is the free-sliding layers of fascia surrounding these organs, like greasy plastic wrap, that enables them to do this.

Any reduction in a body's water content will adversely affect the fascia. It becomes more viscous, or gel-like. It becomes sticky and starts to stick to itself and other structures in the body. This process effectively squeezes the water out of the fascia and the tissues it supports. Communication between the cells reduces and toxins build up in the tissues as their normal transport system has ceased to work.

Even a temporary 2% reduction in your water balance will significantly affect how your body functions. Many people are almost permanently dehydrated as a diet of processed foods, drinks, alcohol, and caffeine either does not deliver enough water to the body, or acts as a diuretic to speed the increased release of water out of the body.

How much water you drink affects how well your fascia works.

How fascia behaves

A knowledge of how fascia behaves is the key to harnessing the power of fascia in the treatment of chronic pain, whether it is treatment by a fascial therapist or self-help treatment using the techniques and exercises in this book. We have already seen how fascia adapts to accommodate other physical structures around it. Now let us consider the properties of fascia itself.

Movement and balance (tensegrity)

At this point you would be forgiven for assuming that this elegant, fragile-looking tissue is weak, but do not be fooled. Fascia has a tensile strength of 2,000 lb per square inch (roughly equivalent to the force of a panda sitting on you!). It is this fascial strength that holds the body together, maintaining its shape and enabling movement.

Within the body, fascia creates a structure that is perfectly balanced, strong and flexible, and able to adjust to changes in tension without

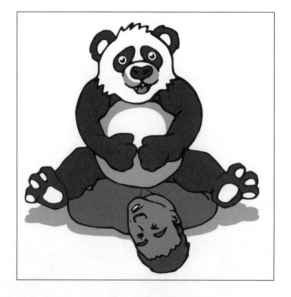

Figure 5.4: Fascia has a tensile strength of 2,000 lb per square inch – imagine the force of a panda sitting on you!

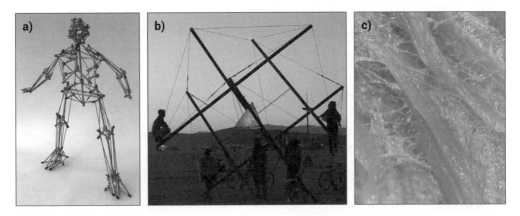

Figure 5.5: Examples of tensegrity structures (a & b) compared with an image of fascia (c, courtesy of Julian Baker).

losing its structure. In architecture this is known as tensegrity. Tensegrity structures offer the maximum strength for any given amount of material. Tensegrity is what enables suspension bridges and skyscrapers to defy the forces of gravity and wind to remain standing. From nature we might think of a tree growing twisted or straight, adjusting to its environment.

Returning briefly to the traditional anatomical view of the body, this says that structure is provided by the skeleton, and the bones are the load-bearing structures in the body. However, in fascial anatomy it is the tensegrity of fascia that provides structure and the bones are anchor points within the fascial web. Without fascia, the living skeleton would be no more than a pile of bones on the floor.

An image often referred to in the world of fascia research is that if you removed every other structure in the body except for the fascia, you would be left with a perfect three-dimensional representation of a person, right down to facial expression.

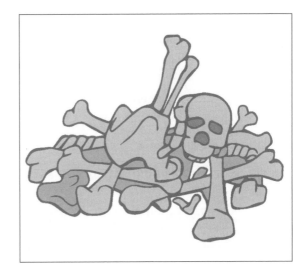

Figure 5.6: Without fascia we would be nothing more than a pile of bones on the floor.

No wonder Robert Schleip has called fascia the Cinderella tissue that has been overlooked for too long.

Resistance and giving (thixotrophy)

The tensegrity of fascia gives it strength and structure. Its high water content gives it another quality related to bounce and give.

The protein mesh that binds water into fascia gives fascia a trampoline-like ability to yield and bounce. This is called viscoelasticity. The combination of water and protein in fascia has a gel-like consistency with a property called thixotrophy.

Thixotrophy is the ability to change consistency quite dramatically and move from gel to fluid, and gel to more solid matter. Thixotrophy is triggered by temperature (heat) and mechanical force (pressure). If you subject a thixotrophic substance to a short sharp shock it will immediately resist and harden but if you apply gentle sustained pressure it will "melt" and become fluid.

Thixotrophy helps to explain why the trauma of forceful injury, such as accident or surgery, can cause fascia to solidify and get stuck (leading to problems); and how stuck fascia can be released using the warm gentle pressure of a hands-on fascial therapy such as myofascial release.

Between these two extremes, thixotrophy and certain other qualities of proteins also explain how over-use over a sustained period can lead to a thickening and solidifying of fascia, and to repetitive strain injuries and chronic conditions. Again, it also helps to explain how myofascial release can successfully treat these conditions. We will talk more about this in Chapter 8.

Fascia as a communication system

The idea of fascia as a communication system works on two levels:

- fascia as a physical web able to conduct the forces required for movement
- fascia as a communication network able to transmit messages.

Fascia contains more nerve endings than any other tissue. This makes fascia incredibly sensitive to change and also gives it the potential to communicate change throughout the body.

Most of the nerve endings associated with proprioception are contained in the fascia. Proprioception is the very practical ability to sense where we are in relation to other things. Damage to fascia can cause our proprioception to become distorted so we can become clumsy or susceptible to injury. This usually affects a particular area or one side of our body more than the other. If you have ever had your arm in a sling and yet still managed to bash it on the refrigerator door, or kept going over on the same ankle, you will know what I mean.

Many fascia therapists and researchers believe that the sensitivity of fascia is the source of our mysterious "sixth sense" – that feeling we have when we are out of sorts and just know something is not quite right. As the gut is made almost entirely of fascia, it is no coincidence that it is where we experience that form of knowledge we call our "gut feeling."

It is human experiences such as these that have led fascial researchers to propose that fascia is a communication system in its own right – one that works faster than the nervous system to communicate feelings before they are registered consciously and to coordinate the body's response to messages.

We will see why this is important later in our discussion about how chronic pain develops. In the meantime, let us just remind ourselves of Andrew Taylor Still's description of fascia as the branch offices of the brain, and D. D. Palmer's belief in an intelligent thinking system, connecting and unifying the functions of the brain and the body, and essential to health.

Fascia and the extracellular matrix (ECM)

What makes fascia such a fascinating subject for modern holistic and scientific study are the many levels on which its real physical structure and qualities are related to many human body–mind experiences.

Going back to traditional anatomy, you will recall that our cells all exist bathed in a fluid that carries nutrients to them and waste from them. This fluid is known by various names, one of which is the extracellular matrix (ECM), the complex substance outside cells.

ECM is the most fluid form of fascia. It has a sieve-like structure that affects everything passing through it. In one way or another every communication within the body travels through the ECM and therefore through the fascial system.

- ECM forms an essential part of the immune system barrier keeping our cells healthy.
- From an evolutionary point of view (remember when we were just single-celled blobs?), the ECM is older than the hormonal or nervous systems, and can communicate more effectively than either, as electrical messages are conducted through water at great speed.
- ECM acts as a physical shock-absorber, lubricating our joints.
- ECM controls all movement in the body by sending messages to and from muscles and bones.
- Malfunctions in ECM are the cause of chronic and systemic diseases, such as rheumatism, fibromyalgia, and even cancer.

One of the most thorough examinations of ECM was done by Austrian researcher Alfred Pischinger, who was the first scientist to start to research and describe this fascinating substance back in the 1940s.

Pischinger demonstrated that ECM has a direct two-way connection with the brain and established that all disease and illness derives from a lack of balance in ECM regulation.

In all diseases and illnesses, whether physical or psychological, acute or chronic, the structure of ECM changes. And ECM is particularly vital to our understanding of systemic inflammatory conditions such as fibromyalgia and rheumatoid arthritis, both of which are both difficult to understand and difficult to treat effectively with medical methods.

Dehydration can lead to ECM becoming sticky and waste products and toxins can become trapped instead of passing out of the body. This causes cells to react and inflammation to occur. Over time this can lead to the development of tumors and to the apparently sudden onset of allergies. This can all be exacerbated by psychological stresses.

It is the accumulation of imbalances in the ECM that frequently leads to the development of chronic conditions in the over 50s. By this age, our systems reach the limit of their tolerance and illness can be triggered by a stressful event – physical, chemical or emotional.

The flip side of this is that the release of imbalances within the fascial system can offer effective healing for systemic disease and chronic conditions.

Fascia and energy

We saw in Chapter 4 that modern quantum physicists have proved that the world is made of energy. Even those things we think of as solid matter are made solid only by the energy holding them together.

We have also noted how electrical energy can be conducted through the watery content of fascia, but there is another way in which fascia holds and releases energy which is also related to its high water content.

The watery electrical nature of fascia means that it is highly sensitive to electrical and magnetic changes, such as changes in the weather. People who experience headaches before a thunderstorm, or an achy knee before it rains, have developed more than normal sensitivity in their fascia.

The water held in cells and fascia is a special form of water called "bound water." Bound water is denser than normal water. This density gives desert plants the ability to retain moisture even in extremely arid conditions and animals the ability to survive in arctic conditions as bound water freezes at much lower temperatures than fluid water.

When fascia lets go of its bound water, energy in the form of electricity is released. This enables movement to occur and communicates change.

Fascial memory

One form of memory is held in the brain (see Chapter 7). Another form of memory, alluded to in the quote from Andrew Taylor Still at the beginning of this chapter, is tissue memory. Tissue memory can explain why "practice makes perfect."

From Taylor Still's fascial perspective, memory is held in the fascia, the branch offices of the brain. Sports people, ballet dancers, and musicians all use this aspect of fascia to improve their performance. Using the fluidity of fascia, repetition of movement and conscious thought to improve tissue memory, they can perform complex virtuoso movements and make them appear instinctual. Many elite athletes and musicians refine and enhance their specialism by imagining their performance, as the mind–body connection means there is no difference between actual and imagined actions – both reinforce tissue memory.

Beyond the world of elite performance an understanding of fascia has the potential to inform occupational health, holistic therapies, and self-healing.

What does this mean for fascia, injury, and disease?

* fascia is a three-dimensional web that, in more or less solid form, runs throughout the body, maintaining structure and health.
* fascia is a communication network that conducts physical forces and communicates chemical and electrical messages to body tissues.
* injury and imbalances in the fascia create the conditions for disease.
* an understanding of the fascial system offers us new ways to treat injury, disease, and chronic pain conditions.

CHAPTER
6

Injury and Fascia

Stress is defined as the body's non-specific response to any demand made upon it.

Hans Selye, stress researcher

In this chapter we will recap some fascial anatomy and discover:

- what happens when fascia is injured or damaged
- the consequences of fascial restrictions over time
- the particular effects of overuse and underuse on health and healing.

Introduction

We saw in Chapter 5 how, in its natural state, fascia is a complex three-dimensional web of free-moving structural tissue that constantly shapes and reshapes itself in response to our movements and the demands we make on it. In its healthy state, fascia moves fluidly and seamlessly to distribute tension and maintain balance in the body.

However, like every other part of us, fascia can suffer accident or injury or be damaged in some other way, for example by surgery. When this happens the fascial web can snag, become misshapen, and lose its flexibility and ability to move. This causes fascial restrictions, and it is these fascial restrictions that lead to limited movement, pressure, and pain. Other major causes of fascial damage and restrictions are the overuse and underuse of our bodies associated with modern lifestyles, and psychological stress and trauma.

Before we look at the causes of fascial injury and restriction, let us talk in more detail about how injury affects fascia.

How injury affects fascia

According to Robert Schleip, fascia is one interconnected tensional network that adapts its fiber arrangement and density according to local tensional demands. In other words, fascia constantly changes and adapts to whatever pressures are put on it.

Any damage to fascia causes it to snag and tear, pulling the web out of shape, similar to a snag in a jumper or a pair of tights.

Fascia contains special cells called fibroblasts that are responsible for maintaining its structure. When any damage occurs to the fascia, the fibroblasts are stimulated into producing collagen, the strong structural protein, to repair the damage. In many cases, the fibroblasts complete the repair and the fascial web returns to normal balanced function.

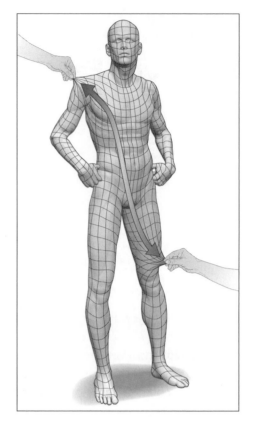

Figure 6.1: Strain in one area of the fascial web can be transmitted elsewhere in the body.
(Illustration reproduced from Massage Fusion *(Fairweather and Mari, 2015) with permission from Handspring Publishing).*

However, there are also many occasions when the damage creates increased tension in the fascia around the injury. This tension triggers the fibroblasts to keep producing more collagen as they repeatedly try to repair the damage.

Over time this extra collagen creates adhesions (where the fascia sticks to itself and other tissues), thickening of the fascia (called fibrosis), and a reduction in the fascia's ability to slide freely. This can turn into a vicious cycle in which the body continues to produce more collagen, which creates more "stuckness" and irritation of the fascia, which stimulates more collagen production.

As the extra collagen forms it also starts to squeeze the fluid out of the fascia. Remembering thixotrophy (see previous chapter), this changes the damaged fascia from fluid to gel and eventually to a solid tissue no longer capable of fluid free movement. As fascia in its natural state is formed of 70% water, this is a bit like squeezing the water out of a sponge. This changes the sponge, or tissue, from being soft and pliable to being hard and brittle in texture. Everything contained within the dehydrated fascia, including muscles, nerves, and blood vessels, is squeezed to the point that it cannot relax and let go.

At first the fascial tension is limited to the original area of damage but over time this spreads and starts to affect adjoining areas and then to create more widespread changes as the lines of tension throughout the body alter. At this stage fascial tension can cause changed muscle tone, a loss of coordination, and imbalanced posture where one side is favored more than the other. Over time this creates a change to the balance of the whole body structure.

Fascial tension also stimulates the nerve endings that measure damage and signal pain. This increased activity further stimulates yet more production of collagen and a tendency for the body to stop using the area it thinks is still damaged – we become "protective" of our injuries.

A long-term result of untreated fascial tension is physical change in the nervous system, called central sensitization. We will look at this in more detail in Chapter 7, because it is these changes that lead to the development of chronic pain conditions.

In addition to the physical adaptations that occur in fascia as a result of damage, the tissue memory (sometimes called somatic recall) that we discussed in Chapter 5 comes into play. Research in this area is ongoing but suggests that the memory of everything that happens to our bodies is not just stored in the brain, but is also held locally in the fascia. These memories are held as energy within the stuck fascial tissue. Your body is literally holding on tight.

This explains why holistic hands-on therapists often find that touching an area, or releasing physical tension can trigger an emotional response. Flashback memory can also occur as a long-forgotten event suddenly floods back. Often the discharge of this memory releases the physical tissue restriction and resolves the pain.

In my work with clients I have experienced this many times. Without expecting it, someone suddenly experiences a surge of anxiety as they relive an accident or recall an injury from 20 years ago. In all cases, as the anxiety quickly peaks and falls away, the memories and emotions are effectively released from their tissues and people report an associated reduction in pain and an increase in energy levels.

We will discuss more about the relationship between pain and emotion in Chapter 7.

How injury to fascia occurs

Accident

All of us will experience a variety of accidents and injuries during our lives, from childhood through to old age. You may immediately have thought of something, such as a car crash, breaking a leg, or similar. A major trauma will usually be remembered long after the event and can have long-lasting effects. These effects may be apparent in the weeks and months after an accident but they can also emerge years later, having been carried in the fascia long after superficial healing takes place, whether or not you have obvious scars. (Please see below for scar tissue.)

Even those everyday minor incidents, such as bumping into a kitchen cupboard, missing your footing as you step off a kerb, or stubbing your toe, can create fascial injuries that are communicated deeper into the body. What may soon be forgotten by the conscious mind stays with us and can have consequences later in life.

Both major and minor accidents are relatively high-impact compared with other forms of injury to fascia and both are likely to cause snagging and tearing. These snags and tears, and the healing processes that take place around them, create imbalances and fresh lines of tension within the body that pull on surrounding areas, causing physical and other problems.

For example, if you are involved in a car accident you may experience whiplash, a soft tissue injury that occurs when your head is suddenly jolted forward and then back. Whiplash damages the fascia in your neck and shoulders. As more collagen fibers are created to patch and strengthen the tears, restrictions develop.

These restrictions create stiffness that limits movement and abnormal tensions result in further issues. For one person the consequence could be headaches and for another it might be lower back pain.

There is another aspect to high-impact fascial injuries, and that relates to energy. Again taking the example of a car crash, in addition to creating visual and other memories, the high impact of the event causes energy to become stuck in the fascia in the form of tissue memory which then becomes associated with emotion.

Through the mechanisms we will describe in Chapter 7, the immediate pain of an accident and unresolved damage to fascia can lead to chronic pain.

How well our fascia heals after an accident depends partly on how healthy it was to start with and partly on how we treat it afterwards. That is why an understanding of fascial anatomy and the energetic properties of fascia is so important in treatment and self-help after accidents.

Surgery and scar tissue

Hundreds of millions of surgical procedures take place every year. These can be emergency surgery to save a life after an accident or to remove an infected organ (an appendix, for example), or necessary planned surgery to remove a cancerous growth. Roughly one in every four pregnancies in the UK results in a Caesarian section at childbirth.

Some people voluntarily undergo cosmetic surgery to refine their visual appearance by facelift or liposuction. Dental work is a good example of surgery that can be cosmetic or essential, partly depending on your point of view.

Whether it is major or minor, voluntary or involuntary, necessary or not, all surgery creates scar tissue. In the case of people who have surgery after an accident this can be scar tissue on top of scar tissue, and in those who have repeated surgery this leads to layers and layers of accumulated scar tissue, some of which will be surface and much of which is held deep within the body.

Surface scarring, particularly minor scarring, may heal and disappear as the surrounding area returns to normal. In other cases, the scars remain, looking and feeling different from the surrounding tissues.

Bigger scars are multi-layered – what you see and feel on the surface of your skin is the tip of the fascial iceberg. Unseen, under the surface of the skin, it is very common for these scars to expand, growing along lines of fascial tension and creating adhesions (as discussed above). These adhesions can cause obstructions and problems of their own. They can block other organs, limit movement and function, and compress nerves, contributing to the development of chronic pain.

Sometimes these problems can be so extreme a surgeon may suggest operating again to remove the adhesions, and so the cycle begins again.

Overuse and underuse

As fluid beings, we are designed to move and to use our bodies. However, as our world has become more advanced, systems, machines, and gadgets have been invented that have changed our lifestyles and how we move.

Overuse and underuse are related and growing problems arising from our modern lifestyles, including work and leisure. Both cause fascial injuries.

Most people actually subject their bodies to a powerful combination of underuse and overuse that can almost be characterized as abuse.

There is barely a client I see who does not, in some way, attribute the physical (and mental) stress they feel and the problems they experience to the work they do. Similarly, very few see exercise as a problem. But things are rarely as simple as that. For some of us, work is the only physical activity we do. If we did not work we would be in a worse state. For others the problem is the intensity with which we pursue our leisure activities, whether in the gym or with the X-box.

The following examples will be recognizable to many, but it is important not to fall for stereotypes. Damaging overuse can happen in everyday situations if our job demands that we do any limited action repeatedly for long periods. Equally, underuse can be just as damaging. And we may do more damage to ourselves outside work than in it.

The important thing is to start to gain an understanding of the demands that any activity or inactivity makes on our fascia.

Work

According the World Health Organization, most of us will spend at least one-third of our life at work, and work is a dangerous place to be! Some of us work in arduous physical industries where better health and safety is needed to reduce the risk of accident, while others are at risk of "ergonomic injuries" that demand better awareness of occupational health.

Ergonomic injuries affect those of us who do manual work and those of us who work in an office. In both contexts our work has become more specialized and the need to move has been reduced. This process has been affecting ever greater numbers of people since the early days of industrial revolution.

Previously, many traditional forms of manual labor required great strength and flexibility. People were required to continually move their bodies in different directions and with varying degrees of force. As jobs became more mechanized this need lessened. In factories, production lines developed. These again reduced the need to move, because now the work came to you, and divided previously whole-istic jobs into ever smaller specialized tasks requiring a reduced repertoire of movement. We have now reached the stage where robots may do the production line work while we sit in a control room, staring at a computer screen.

In offices, the process has been similar. In the typing pools of the 1950s and 1960s, the women (as it generally was) who operated manual typewriters worked in a highly organized environment but still had a certain degree of movement in their work. They needed to use force to press the typewriter keys and shoulder movement to operate the carriage return at the end of every line. As they finished each typed sheet, the paper would need to be changed and this provided an opportunity to roll and stretch their shoulders. Every so often they would get up to deliver their work to a central collection point and to pick up more.

In modern offices we now operate ever decreasing sizes of keyboard that require minimal movement of our hands and fingers. And we hunch over for hours on end, stuck in one position, staring at our computer screen. The need to get up and physically move to talk to colleagues has been replaced by email and instant messaging.

All of this has an effect on our fascia. For as long as we keep moving our fascia remains fluid. But if we stay in one position for more than 2 minutes (yes, 2 *minutes!*), our body thinks we want to make a permanent change and starts to lay down new fascia to help with this. At this stage this new fascia is a light fuzzy tissue, a bit like fluff or candy floss. If you move normally after a few minutes this candy floss will melt away (remember thixotrophy?) and be reabsorbed. But time spent stuck in one position, hour after hour, day after day, for months and years creates more and more layers of fascia which no longer stay light and fuzzy. The layers start to stick together like Velcro, and harden, eventually becoming like plywood.

This is underuse in action. We are not moving enough to keep our body mobile. The impact of this is far reaching. Over time our muscles become less able to stretch and may even start to calcify (turn to bone), bones become harder and more brittle, nerves, blood vessels, and organs are literally squeezed to the point that they no longer function properly.

At the same time as underuse, our work situations often create overuse of specific parts of the body. For example, working at a computer for many hours, day in day out, involves chronic overuse of the muscles and fascia in our forearms and hands. None of these muscles are particularly big, which means it does not take much to tire them. However, if we keep typing and using our mouse, we overuse these muscles and irritate them to the point of damage, as the fascia that surrounds them becomes stuck into one big irritated lump of tissue.

If you recall from Chapter 5 the need for our fascia to remain fluid and free-moving to shift and accommodate our organs you will appreciate why the underuse and overuse exemplified by the western "sitting epidemic" has become a major issue resulting in all sorts of problems, including digestive and respiratory ones.

Leisure
We may not have appreciated the depth of the physical effects that can come from underuse but many of us are ("painfully") aware that sitting immobile for hours does not burn up many calories. To counteract this, we may spend our spare time frantically jogging, swimming, or at the gym.

Without fascial awareness, far from providing the antidote to work, these activities can exacerbate problems. Just imagine the shock that an underused body experiences going from hours of underuse to short bursts of high-intensity activity, particularly when most of us are careless with our warm-up and warm-down routines, use equipment incorrectly, and, if we run, run on hard unforgiving surfaces. But not just that.

Our bodies work on a "use it or lose it" principle. It is quite likely that by the time we decide we need more exercise in our life we will have lost the fitness we are seeking through underuse. It is possible to get it back and this is the physiological principle on which all training is based. If you want bigger muscles, lift weights. By doing so your body sends fascial messages to your brain telling it to create more muscle fibers to add bulk. Likewise, if it is flexibility you want, do more yoga and your fascia and muscles will respond by adding length. (See Chapter 11 for more on fascial stretching techniques for particular injuries and pain conditions.)

However, it is possible to overdo physical exercise, and this results in overuse injuries. Often these overuse injuries occur in sports-specific training when we repeat the same actions over and over. Using one set of muscles repetitively will fatigue the tissues and cause fascial injuries. If our body is not used to the repetition, we pile on tension that exacerbates weaknesses, creates imbalances, and results in restrictions.

Even when we are not pulled up by a sudden "pulled muscle," overuse creates micro tears in the tissues, like tiny scars, that can build up and harden and develop into adhesions. Runner's knee, golfer's elbow, tennis elbow are all overuse injuries that can be understood and treated fascially.

Exercise has many mind–body benefits and I am not saying that we must stop exercising, but I am asking everyone to consider doing so with a new appreciation of their fascia.

It is better to exercise than not – but to avoid injury do it paying attention to the fascia.

Posture

Most adults have some kind of postural imbalance that has developed as a result of their work, leisure activities, and, to a certain extent, family habits.

Next time you are with members of your family (or your partner's family), look at how they all hold themselves when they sit or stand. As you observe them, you'll start to see that not only do they look alike, but they typically sit or stand in a similar way. This is not genetics, it is a familial learned behavior, and it can lead to families passing on apparently inherited conditions such as bad backs or headaches.

When functioning properly, the body is held upright by ligaments and fascia rather than by muscles. It can maintain an upright position without conscious postural control or muscle fatigue. This is tensegrity (see Chapter 5) in action, the same principle that keeps a suspension bridge suspended.

Say we sit at a desk for long periods, this is an unnatural posture held for an unnaturally long time. Our fascia tightens to maintain this position, exerting new forces within our body. This causes the fascia to become less fluid and more rigid, effectively forming a type of scar tissue.

Poor posture at your desk is likely to result in muscle fatigue and in neck pain causing inflammation. In an unconscious (and sometimes conscious) effort to alleviate the neck pain we tend to adjust our posture, which leads to a vicious cycle of restricted movement and thickened fascia. Eventually we can end up literally stuck in a slumped posture with a stiff and painful neck.

What started as a pain in your neck can become back pain or a frozen shoulder. If the fascial restrictions affect the vagus nerve (literally the "wandering nerve" that starts from the neck and wanders through the body), this can also affect hearing, speech and swallowing, heart rate and blood pressure, breathing, digestive function, and bladder control. As the vagus nerve is also involved with controlling inflammation, systemic conditions such as fibromyalgia or myofascial pain syndrome can also develop. These can all be understood and treated myofascially.

In their anatomical dissection research many researchers, including the Steccos and Tom Myers (see Chapter 5), have demonstrated these thickened lines of fascia and how to read the stories of posture they tell.

Ask a work colleague or a friend to take a photo, or even better a video, of you using a computer. Tell them to wait until you are absorbed in whatever you are doing otherwise you will consciously correct your posture. When they are done, take a look at the result. Look at the position of your head, neck, shoulders, and so on. Without even having met you, I will guess that your head is strained forward, your shoulders are rounded and slumped. This is called "forward head position," which is an unnatural position held in the fascia.

Stress

Stress can be both physical and mental.

As we have seen in Chapter 5, stress is a natural phenomenon and a physiological response to both real and perceived danger. Some stress can be good. Running to avoid a speeding car as you cross the road can save your life. The stress of a virus entering your system will trigger your immune system to kick in and resolve the temporary illness, which is a good thing.

But after just 7 days of sustained increased stress, the mind–body goes into a state of exhaustion in which normal protective immune responses are no longer triggered and the body is vulnerable to disease and injury.

The everyday effects of stress

Stress is a natural part of everyday life, but most people now only associate with the negative aspects of it. People often have guilt and shame around stress: they reproach themselves for not being able to cope better. At the same time they accept that they are "stressed" as a catch-all explanation for their apparent inability to cope with everyday situations.

The problem with stress in our modern society is not actually our reaction to it, but rather the frequency with which it occurs and the lack of control we have over it. Rather than being exposed to a single major event, we are bombarded with minor stressful situations every day, from the alarm that jolts us out of sleep to getting stuck in traffic, working to tight deadlines, or repeatedly receiving nuisance calls.

Any one of these situations is a temporary stressor, but if these things happen frequently enough they can grind down our stress resistance and accumulate to the point that our mind–body is too exhausted to fight off illness. In other words, the more we have to deal with, the less efficient at coping our mind–body becomes, so the more quickly we become exhausted until eventually just one small thing can tip our overloaded system into illness.

Previously stress-related illnesses tended to appear in the over 50s, categorized as a "nervous breakdown," but the increasingly stressful nature of modern life explains why these illnesses are appearing in much younger people. It also explains the increasing incidence of systemic-type conditions such as fibromyalgia, chronic fatigue, and myofascial pain syndrome, where the whole mind–body system just rolls over onto its back and gives up.

Stress and the digestive system

Chronic stress has a particularly strong impact on the digestive system. This system is at the frontline of interaction with the external environment as it processes everything that we eat and drink. Not only that, but it also plays a crucial role in maintaining our overall mind–body balance, as it continually exchanges information with the brain via the vagus nerve.

The level to which the digestive system can function is dependent on our stress levels. Because our stress system originally evolved to keep us safe from danger, it effectively shuts down "non-essential" parts of the body in stressful situations. The shut-down includes our digestive system – which is why when we are nervous we tend to feel sick or go right off our food.

If the digestion is chronically under pressure because the whole of the mind–body is out of balance, then it too will lose balance and with it the ability to effectively absorb the nutrients and minerals we need, and dispose of the toxins and waste products that we do not need.

Not only can this cause digestive illnesses, such as irritable bowel syndrome (IBS) and Crohn's disease, it also causes other more generalized immune system dysfunctions such as allergies, eczema, and autoimmune diseases.

A poorly functioning digestive system also affects the function of the vagus nerve, affecting many vital body responses such as speech, breathing, heart rate, and liver function.

The stress–pain cycle

Any physical pain, whether it is the initial damage caused by an accident or the chronic irritation of overused muscles and fascia, will trigger the stress response. Initially this is a good thing, causing the body to start the processes needed to repair the damage.

If the damage is resolved, the mind–body returns to normal function and the stress response is switched off. However, as we have seen, there are many times where the mind–body continues to think there is an injury and the fascia is therefore repeatedly triggered to repair it.

Initially the mind–body can cope with these changes, making minute adjustments to tissue consistency and even to posture. However, as the fascia becomes less fluid and more stuck, this puts an additional strain on the whole body and creates a vicious cycle. The ongoing pain caused by the changed tissue texture creates a chronic stress response.

Over time this changes the mind–body from a balanced self-regulating system into an unstable environment where eventually even the slightest additional stress can spread the pain to other areas or magnify it. If you try to ignore it, or you are told "you're just going to have to live with it," this can add just enough stress to tip the original chronic pain into something else.

The stress of ongoing pain also has a degenerative effect on the nervous system, reducing the body's ability to cope with further pain and stress. This can trigger a latent inflammatory response in fascia that ultimately results in the stress-related conditions mentioned above.

Because the mind–body is interlinked, chronic physical pain also creates chronic mental stress. People who have chronic pain are far more likely to suffer from stress-related mental conditions such as anxiety and depression. These too form part of the ongoing stress–pain cycle that maintains many chronic pain conditions (see Chapter 7).

Physical bodywork, such as myofascial release, that works on irritated and stuck fascia can soothe the stress responses, break the vicious cycle, and relieve symptoms.

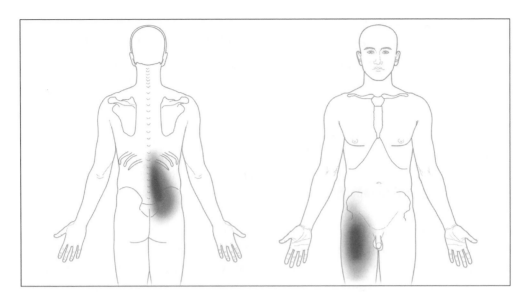

Figure 6.2: A typical referred pain pattern for trigger points in the psoas.

The importance of trigger points

As fascial restrictions develop in the body they cause trigger points to form in areas of tightened or tense tissues.

A trigger point is a distinct area of fascial restriction within the soft tissue. When pressed, a trigger point can feel like anything from a grain of sand to a small golf ball, depending on where it is. Trigger points are what people often call "knots" in their muscles.

When pressed, a trigger point will either produce pain and other symptoms where it is located, or, more typically, refer the pain and symptoms to elsewhere in the body in a specific recognizable pattern.

This is helpful to myofascial therapists. For example, lower back pain can be caused by trigger points in the psoas muscle located in the abdomen. Without necessarily working directly on the lower back, applying gentle sustained pressure to the trigger points in the psoas causes them to release, allowing the pain and other symptoms to subside. This is why myofascial release therapists often work somewhere other than where the pain is felt. This can be useful and reassuring to a client who is anxious about having work done to an area where they are feeling their pain.

Understanding this principle of trigger points and referred pain helps to explain why the self-help exercises we provide in this book do not always work directly where you feel your pain.

The link between fascia and chronic pain

In this chapter we have looked at what happens to fascia when it is injured and what sort of things can happen to cause fascial injury. From this we can see that injury to fascia is intimately involved in the development of chronic pain because:

- injury to fascia changes the whole mind–body balance
- over time, fascial injury changes nervous system function
- chronic pain is a combination of nervous system changes and chronic stress responses in the mind–body.

How Chronic Pain Develops

*[Pain is] an unpleasant sensory and emotional experience associated with
actual or potential tissue damage, or described in terms of such damage.*
The International Association for the Study of Pain (IASP)

In this chapter we will learn:

- how the body's "normal" pain response works
- how this can go wrong, leading the body to get stuck in chronic pain
- what this has to do with fascia.

Introduction

To recap on our understanding of chronic pain (from Chapter 2):

*Chronic pain is defined as pain that persists beyond the normal time
of healing, or occurs in diseases in which healing does not take place.*
Chronic Pain Policy Coalition (CPPC)

We know that chronic pain is pain that persists longer than it should. Before we
can really look at why chronic pain persists we need to look at how and why pain
happens in the first place.

What is pain?

According to the above definition from the International Association for the Study
of Pain, pain is how we perceive it. Say, for example, we are barefoot and we stand

on a sharp stone. First, we sense something out of the ordinary. Second, we create an association and our mind labels it as pain. We have just created an emotional memory to refer back to when we encounter similar events in the future. So the creation of pain is a two-stage body–mind process.

Pain is a necessary and natural response to something potentially damaging. The problems arise when the pain response gets corrupted and turns into an unwanted chronic situation.

The "normal" mind–body pain response (the short version)

The pain response mechanism is shown in Figure 7.1. It is mainly activated and controlled by the nervous system, although there is also some involvement from fascia. The purpose of the pain response is to protect us from something potentially damaging and, if damage occurs, to initiate the repair process.

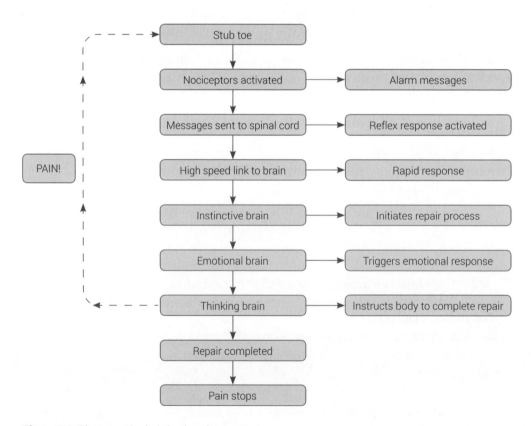

Figure 7.1: The nromal mind–body pain response.

Let us talk through the process. Say we stub our toe on the edge of the bed, the normal pain response mechanism goes like this:

- Nerve receptors located in the fascia, called nociceptors, are squashed by the impact to the toe. Nociceptors are only triggered by abnormal situations where damage occurs and their job is to raise the alarm.
- Nociceptors send their alarm message along nerves that run from the toe to the brain via the spinal cord.
- When the alarm message reaches the spinal cord, it triggers the first protective response, called a reflex response.
- The reflex response is to move your toe away from the bed and out of danger.
- The message continues up the spinal cord via "fast track" fibers that ensure it gets to the brain as quickly as possible because, at this point, the body assumes that any new damage could potentially be life-threatening.
- The message reaches the first area of the brain, the instinctive brain, which is also called the reptilian brain because it is the oldest evolved area.
- The instinctive brain responds by triggering the body to start repairing any damage to the tissues in your toe. It also sets in motion a number of unconscious body-wide reactions that we shall look at in more detail below. They are all designed to keep you safe from further danger.
- The alarm message continues up to the next area of your brain, called the emotional or limbic brain.
- The emotional brain responds by creating a basic initial emotional response, which may be anger, fear, tears, or something else. The emotion it chooses is unique to you and depends on your personal library of stored emotions.
- The alarm message continues up to the final area of your brain, called the thinking brain, or cortex.
- It is only when the alarm message reaches the thinking brain that the message is first interpreted as pain. This is when you become consciously aware of it. Although this conscious awareness happens within a split second of the original damage, already a whole set of unconscious responses have been triggered.
- The thinking brain will now run a quick scan of its stored memories to see if it has a match to this current situation.
- If it finds a match, it will also retrieve an associated emotion, as the brain catalogs memories keeping the emotions attached (a bit like attaching a note to the front of a file). The thinking brain will then instruct the emotional brain to run that emotion.
- If it cannot find a match, the thinking brain will create a new memory and associated emotion and store these together for future reference. The emotion it selects will relate to the circumstances around you stubbing your toe.

For example, if you stubbed your toe in the middle of an argument with your partner, the brain would store the emotion of the argument with the memory of toe stubbing.

- From now on, when you stub your toe this emotion will drive your reaction.
- The thinking brain is also responsible for instructing the body to complete the repair to the injury.
- As part of this process it will send a flood of pain-killing chemicals back down the spinal cord. This is why often people do not feel much pain when they first injure themselves.
- After a while these pain killing chemicals run out. At this point pain enhancing chemicals take over; these are designed to make you stop using the injured area while it heals.
- In the normal course of events, the body completes its repair, the nociceptors (from step 1) calm down, and your body returns to normal day-to-day activities.
- The pain stops.

When pain becomes chronic (the short version)

The chronic pain response mechanism is shown in Figure 7.2. Based on our previous example of stubbing your toe on the bed, sometimes the repair process goes wrong, as follows:

- In the process of repairing the damage to your toe, the fascia in the area may start to add extra collagen to patch the damage, as this is fascia's response to getting injured (see Chapter 6). Although the body completes its repair, the thickened fascia has now lost some of its sliding ability, which means the tissues cannot return to their pre-injury state.
- As a result the nociceptors in this area remain squashed and continue to send their alarm messages to the brain via the spinal cord.
- After only a few days of fascial restriction the number of nociceptors in the area will double, which means they can now send double the number of alarm messages.
- The nociceptors are now also much more sensitive to the possibility of further damage, so they will sometimes spontaneously trigger for no reason, a bit like a false start in a race.
- However, because these messages are no longer "new" news, and are now recognized as not being life-threatening, they are downgraded to the "slow fibers" in the spinal cord. They just become a bit of a nag.

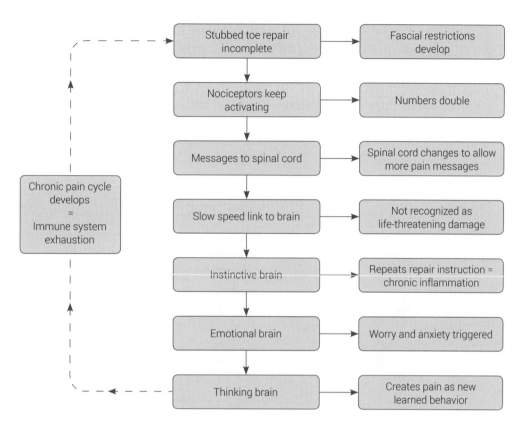

Figure 7.2: When pain becomes chronic.

- On their way up the spinal cord, these nagging messages still pass through the instinctive brain and the emotional brain to reach the thinking brain.
- Now traveling at a slower speed, and moving in a continual wave, the alarm messages have more time to trigger responses in the instinctive and emotional areas of the brain. In particular, they repeatedly trigger the release of stress hormones and emotions associated with stress, such as anxiety and depression.
- As the messages reach the thinking brain they trigger the toe stubbing emotion as well, over and over.
- In time the repetition of this emotional memory reinforces anger (or whatever the original emotion was) as a new way of being, a learned behavior. In this way our mind–body learns chronic pain and an associated emotion.
- The repeated alarm messages from toe to brain also physically change the spinal cord so that instead of pain-killing chemicals, it now transmits only pain-enhancing chemicals. The chronic pain message is continually strengthened.

- This process is called sensitization. Sensitization creates body-wide changes, including exhaustion of the immune system and an increased sensitivity to further pain, which are characteristic of chronic pain.
- The chronic pain causes us to use our body differently, as the injured fascia creates further restrictions which spread along new lines of tension. This alters our balance and posture and may cause yet more pain.
- At the same time, our emotions change because of the pain, which makes us less tolerant to many things. We become short-tempered, which makes us more anxious and depressed.
- We have now entered a chronic pain cycle.

For many readers this explanation of pain and how it can become chronic will be sufficient. If you prefer, you can skip the next section and go straight to Chapter 8, where we look at how to get ourselves out of this chronic pain cycle.

If you would like more detail about the chronic pain cycle then read on.

The "normal" mind–body pain response (the long version)

In this section we will look in more detail at the structures and processes involved in creating normal pain.

Nerve endings and receptors

There are no dedicated pain sensors in the body, just sensors whose job it is to pick up the different changes that can happen to a body. These sensors are called nerve endings.

All body tissues contain millions of embedded nerve endings and each of these has a highly specialized role detecting a specific stimulant. Some exist to detect heat or cold, some detect soft brushing pressure, some detect hard sustained pressure, some give us our sense of proprioception (where we are physically in relation to other things). Importantly for our understanding of pain, there are some sensors that detect the presence of something harmful. This can include, for example, chemicals, heat, pressure, injury, or irritation.

These sensors are called nociceptors ("*noci*" meaning to harm – remember the nocebo effect?) and there are 10 times more of them in fascia than any other tissue in the body. This means that any potential damage to the body is always detected by a combination of the fascial system and nervous system working together.

> If you want to feel your nociceptors in action, tap your fingers on a hard surface. If you tap lightly, you will just feel the pressure of the surface. If you tap harder, you may start to notice the sensation of slight pain, which means that you have just woken up the nociceptors in your fingertips.

Nociceptors do not respond to normal day-to-day events. They respond only to something out of the ordinary, or when conditions go from being normal to being harmful. A nociceptor will not respond to us moving around and exercising as normal, but it will respond if we overstretch a muscle or joint or twist an ankle.

A nociceptor's job is to pick up information about harmful conditions and communicate it to the brain so the brain can act on the information and keep us safe.

The brain

The brain is a 3 lb lump of soft nervous tissue located in the skull.

The brain is the body's nerve control center, receiving and processing messages from nerve receptors and the fascial system all over the body. The brain is responsible for our memory, emotions, balance, and vital unconscious functions such as breathing and circulation.

The brain is made of different parts, which have evolved at different times, as the human species has evolved. The oldest part of our brain (the instinctive brain) controls the vital unconscious functions that keep us alive; the second part of our brain is the emotional brain and deals with emotion. The more modern part of our brain is the thinking and memory part, the cortex. If we go back to our diagram of the normal pain response (see Figure 7.1), we will see that all of these parts of the brain are involved in the pain response.

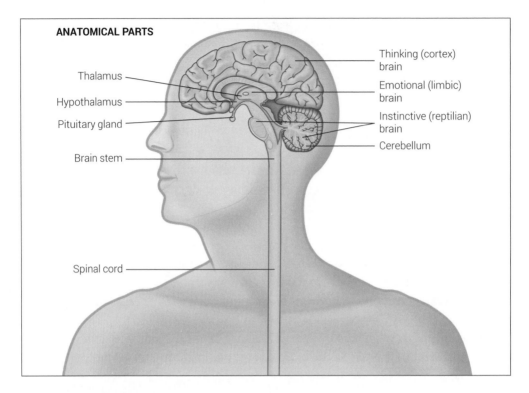

Figure 7.3: The brain is made of different parts, which have evolved at different times, as the human species has evolved.

The brain and the mind compared

Unlike the brain, which is made of physical matter, the mind is something more ethereal. The mind does not exist in solid physical form but consists of the energy that flows through the brain in the form of electrical messages.

Holistically, the brain and mind are intimately interconnected as the processes that occur in the mind can only happen through the physical wires and contact points in the brain.

The phrase "changing your mind" might help you to get your mind round this concept. You can always change your mind, because it does not exist physically; it is just a mass of electrical charges that can be switched at any time. However, you cannot change your brain unless a physical change is made to the structure, through surgery, drugs, or injury.

When our brains record a new experience, such as new pain, the experience is captured by the firing of a particular arrangement of brain cells, called neurons, which leave them connected for just a few seconds. Through repetition this connection strengthens into a neural pathway, which forms a new memory. Collectively, our neural pathways are how we learn and they become our habits, our go-to reactions in certain situations.

The phrase "neurons that fire together, wire together" is a neat explanation of how this whole process happens.

When we talk about the brain, we mean the physical structure in our head and the neural pathways. But when we talk about the mind, we mean the mental processes that give us the thoughts, memories and emotions we attach to these pathways.

Neurotransmitters

Neurons move messages along neural pathways by passing them in a relay from one cell to the other. Each time a message is passed from cell to cell it has to cross a microscopic gap, or synapse. The messages are carried across the gap by neurotransmitters.

Neurotransmitters are natural chemical communicators which switch body functions on or off and there are many different types, some of which you may have heard of (Table 7.1).

Table 7.1 lists the neurotransmitters and chemicals involved in pain. Several of these are actually the "good guys," chemicals that make us feel better and which create an important modulating response when we first feel pain. Some are pain chemicals that act to communicate and to enhance pain, functions vital to keeping us safe.

The normal pain response

Going back to our example of a stubbed toe, an injury such as this causes the local nociceptors to trigger and send alarm messages through the nervous system to the brain. Any tissue damage triggers the release of bradykinin, a pain chemical that stimulates the nociceptors to release another pain chemical called substance P. Substance P is the pain-enhancing chemical that magnifies the alarm signal as it travels up to the brain.

Table 7.1: Chemical neurotransmitters involved in pain and their effects

Chemical neurotransmitter	What it does
Adrenaline (also called epinephrine)	Our "go-faster" chemical
Cortisol	The stress hormone – triggers stress responses
Dopamine	Enhances pleasurable feelings and is involved in addictive behaviors
Serotonin	Enhances pleasurable feelings – a lack of serotonin uptake by the body contributes to depression
Endorphins	The body's natural painkillers which work by blocking the release of substance P (see below)
Enkephalins	Also work to inhibit the release of substance P, and have a painkilling effect 200 times stronger than morphine
Substance P	Enhances the perception of pain and is released in response to injury or damage
Bradykinin	Pain-producing agent first released as a result of tissue damage
Cytokines	The cells' signaling molecules that aid cell to cell communication in immune responses and stimulate the movement of cells towards sites of inflammation, infection, and trauma

As the alarm messages reach the brain they trigger a cascade of actions and associated emotions, as we have seen. Once the brain recognizes the messages as pain, it responds by sending a flood of pain-killing chemicals, such as endorphins and enkephalins, down the spinal cord to dampen the substance P signals that are being sent up by the nociceptors.

In the short term this can mean you feel no pain at first, but then pain will return and intensify as the body exhausts its supply of endorphins and enkephalins although substance P continues to be released.

The brain will also trigger the repair process, encouraging cytokines to signal the area of damage and attract cell repair teams. The initial repair process includes inflammation as a way to prevent you using that part of the body. While you have a swollen toe, you are less likely to walk on it.

Depending on the extent of tissue damage, the repair process can take anything from a few days to weeks to complete, at which point normal tissue function is restored and things return to normal.

The pain is gone.

How normal pain becomes chronic pain

To fully understand how and why normal pain can become chronic pain, we need to understand how fascia can change in response to damage, and how the unconscious systems in our mind–body control our reactions to pain.

The unconscious you

When we talk about the unconscious you, we need to be clear that we are not talking about what happens when you are asleep. What we mean are all of the vital functions that keep us alive without us having to consciously remember to do them. These include things like breathing, our heart beating, digestion, and so on. They also include many of our behaviors, which we may not be aware of but which control how we act in any given situation.

The unconscious you is all powerful, even if you have not been aware of it until now. Our unconscious processes and functions outnumber our conscious thoughts 1 million to one and have already happened before we have even begun to think about getting started. If you think you are in charge of your body, think again!

Figure 7.4 is a diagram of the unconscious nervous system which is divided into three parts:

- brain of the gut
- fight or flight
- rest and digest.

The brain of the gut is the enteric nervous system, which contains five times more neurons than the spinal cord. It works independently of the brain or other parts of the nervous system, although it communicates with the brain via the vagus nerve.

The brain of the gut produces a number of neurotransmitters and is responsible for over 90% of the serotonin and 50% of the dopamine in the body. It also controls all digestive functions.

It is also responsible for our gut reactions, our sixth sense, those unconscious responses to emotional situations where we feel it physically in our gut long before

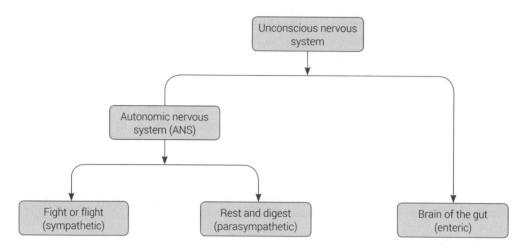

Figure 7.4: The unconscious nervous system.

our mind and reason kick in. Gut reactions usually turn out to be the correct response.

Working in tandem with the brain of the gut are the other two parts of the unconscious nervous system, fight or flight and rest and digest. These are ancient response systems which work in opposition to each other to maintain balance in the body, which is called homeostasis.

The fight or flight response originally evolved to give us the ability to respond to situations of extreme danger, for example being attacked by a saber tooth tiger in prehistoric times. It provides us with the ability to fight the tiger or to run away at speed (flight).

The fight or flight response triggers very specific bodily reactions to prepare you for action. Through the release of adrenaline and cortisol, your breathing and heart rate increase, blood vessels contract to pump oxygen and nutrients to your muscles, your vision becomes more focused and your short-term memory shuts down. Your body also shuts down unnecessary functions such as digestion.

Rest and digest is the exact opposite of the fight or flight response. When this is engaged, your heart and breathing rate slows down, muscles relax and organs such as your stomach and digestive tract start to work normally. This unconscious response is most active when you are asleep.

These two parts of the unconscious are controlled by your instinctive brain. Your instinctive brain will automatically switch between the two responses depending on external and internal triggers, the modern day equivalents of saber tooth tigers. If you are late for work and have to rush to catch the bus, your fight or flight response will kick in to give you the energy to get there. Once you are on the bus and in your seat, your rest and digest response will start to calm you down.

So far so good. But your instinctive brain is not well equipped for the modern world and finds it difficult to distinguish between real danger and perceived danger. So worrying about your job/relationship/money will trigger fight or flight just as a saber tooth tiger or running for the bus will. Stress also triggers fight or flight, as does chronic pain. Constant worry, stress, or pain will all create a repeating cycle of fight or flight.

How good pain turns bad

The main difference between normal pain and chronic pain is that, in chronic pain, the body continues to think there is an injury long after the repair has been completed.

As we know (Chapter 6), fascial restrictions can lead to postural changes and imbalances, and these imbalances sustain chronic pain. Fascial restrictions create a feedback loop between the restricted tissue and the brain. Messages are continually sent around the loop and pain becomes the new normal.

Unconscious responses also contribute to sustaining chronic pain. The pain causes the instinctive brain to repeatedly trigger a fight or flight response because it cannot distinguish between the pain and any other threat. Being in constant fight or flight mode causes chronic stress.

Now you have chronic stress as well as chronic pain. With your whole body in constant fight or flight your muscles remain tense, your heart rate is faster, and your digestion is slower. After a while, your body runs out of energy and becomes exhausted. It can no longer produce adrenaline and cortisol, and you are in adrenal fatigue.

It is likely that all of this pain, stress, and increased activity is affecting your sleep, which means that your body will not be getting the rest and digest time it needs to refuel, repair, and rebuild. Your restricted fascia becomes more restricted, causing more alarm messages to be sent to your brain, piling on the pressure.

On top of this, as your digestion will not be working properly, you will not be producing enough of the feel-good chemicals, dopamine and serotonin, which means you become depressed as well as stressed and in pain. Your mind then responds further by triggering yet more of the worry and anxiety emotions.

You are now in a chronic pain–stress–exhaustion feedback loop.

What this has to do with fascia

As the most widespread and interconnected tissue in the body, fascia is intimately involved in all unconscious processes.

It has more nociceptors than any other tissue, it is more likely to overreact to damage by creating excess repair tissue, and it is more likely to be affected by the stress responses triggered in your brain.

The tightening that happens in your body as part of the fight or flight response happens because of a reaction in your fascia. The natural response of every cell is to contract when faced with a threatening situation. This contraction happens in the fascial web that runs around and through every single cell.

Repeated stress messages cause the fascia to become chronically tight. Remembering the ECM, that essential fluid component of fascia, if fascia is tight some of the fluid gets squeezed out and the remaining fluid becomes unhealthily concentrated with toxins.

Even a 2% reduction in ECM fluid content is enough to cause far reaching changes in the ECM and the fascia.

If the conditions are right (that is, wrong), what started as the inconvenience of stubbing your toe has the potential to develop into a cycle of chronic pain and stress affecting all functions in your body and changing your fascial health in the process.

Therefore, the process of returning to normal pain-free function must start with restoring fascial health. You can begin this through conscious attention to your fascia, fascial self-help exercises, and myofascial release.

What we have learned in this chapter:

- normal pain is a healthy natural process by which the body notices and repairs tissue damage.
- chronic pain develops when fascial repair goes wrong causing body-wide changes.
- the key to returning to normal pain-free function is by restoring fascial health.

What is Myofascial Release?

Myofascial release is a hands-on bodywork technique that works on fascia with a positive understanding of the energies and emotions that shape physical health.

My definition

In this chapter we will learn:

- a little about the hands-on therapy myofascial release (myo + fascia + release) (MFR)
- what myofascial unwinding is and how it works
- how this knowledge can be used to create effective self-help techniques for you to use.

Introduction

We have already seen how many modern anatomy researchers are re-thinking the role of the skeletal system and the muscles in the body. The skeleton is no longer necessarily thought of as the structure that supports the body and from which the muscles hang. And it is the connections between muscles rather than the muscles themselves that drive movement.

Fascia is increasingly recognized as the body's main source of structural support, and the means by which energy and movement is conducted and messages communicated between systems.

Myo + fascia + release

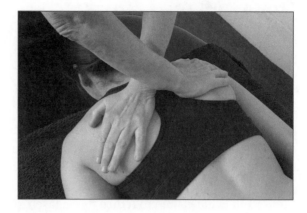

Myo + fascia refers to those new ways of looking at the body. Together, *myo*, meaning muscle, and the fascial web account for almost all of the soft tissue in the human body.

That soft tissue can become damaged, creating snags and restrictions that limit movement and create pain. "Release" refers to the gentle way in which myofascial release works with the

Figure 8.1: Myofascial release is a gentle hands-on therapy working to release the fascial restrictions that cause pain.

natural qualities of fascia to release those snags and restrictions, restoring balance, movement, and health.

As a gentle hands-on therapy that works with the known physical and energetic qualities of fascia, myofascial release (also known as MFR) is an effective holistic treatment option for many types of injury, scar tissue, and chronic pain conditions.

How myofascial release works with fascia

There are three levels on which myofascial release works:

- physical hands-on, to release restrictions in muscle and fascia
- physiological, to relax the nervous system and override pain messages
- emotional, to help the mind–body release the memories and emotions stored as a result of stress and injury.

Myofascial release is a gentle hands-on bodywork technique that works to restore normal movement to the body by releasing restrictions caused by stuck fascia that has become dehydrated and hardened. As the fascia releases, so does the muscle tissue often stuck within it.

These myofascial restrictions can be due to various forms of physical and emotional trauma. In most cases it is a combination of both.

Myofascial release works by the therapist applying gentle and sustained hands-on pressure to the surface of the skin, which is then conducted through the fascia to affect deeper changes. Remembering the property of thixotrophy (see Chapter 5), it is this combination of heat and sustained pressure that returns fascia to its healthy fluid state.

In working in this way a fascial therapist is simply using fascia's natural ability to melt under just the right amount of gentle pressure and heat. On another level, a skilled therapist's hands have been shown scientifically to transmit vibrational piezoelectric energy at the right frequency to encourage natural healing – like a human TENS machine. This vibrational energy encourages restricted tissues to soften, and enables fluid to return to the fascia so that it can relax and move again.

This process relieves abnormal pressure on muscles, bones, nerves, and organs that would otherwise trigger nerve receptors to become active and multiply, and it interrupts the chronic pain cycle.

As well as working to relieve pain responses, myofascial release is effective at breaking down scar tissue. Myofascial release enables excess collagen fibers that build up during healing processes to be reabsorbed or realign with the surrounding tissues and in this way restore more normal flexible movement.

On a physiological level, myofascial release also relaxes the nervous system. There has been much research to prove that the very act of "laying on of hands" can be beneficial if it is done in a caring and empathetic manner. Touch and gentle movement soothes the body and mind and helps to override pain messages. Myofascial touch also engages the rest and digest nervous system and effectively reduces the level of anxiety in pain-sensitive areas.

On an emotional level, myofascial release helps to release and resolve emotional trauma. As we saw in Chapter 7, when the body communicates any unusual physical or mental event to the brain, the thinking brain will store it with an associated emotion. Myofascial release works to release inappropriate stored emotions through "unwinding," which is the process by which the mind–body lets go of physical restrictions and trapped emotions (see below).

With this level of mind–body engagement, myofascial release is more than just a technique, it is an entire therapeutic approach. It has been described as the missing link in healthcare, and as the medicine for the 21st century, explaining and relieving chronic pain and other conditions that have left medical practitioners baffled and unable to offer practical help.

Myofascial unwinding

Myofascial unwinding is a natural process of release by which the mind–body lets go of unwanted physical restrictions and trapped emotions.

Any injury or trauma to the body creates fascial restrictions which, over time, create postural imbalances, holding patterns, and unwanted symptoms and behaviors. Connected to these are the stored emotions that accompanied the original accident or circumstance that is at the root of the problem.

The level on which myofascial unwinding works differs from person to person, depending less on their actual physical pain and more on the willingness of their mind–body to let go of old holding patterns, habits, postures, and emotions, all of which contribute to their current symptoms. The ability to let go is not so much a conscious effort but more an unconscious event that gives the mind and body space to release and repair.

The holding patterns that develop from fascial restrictions are learned behaviors, and as these are unlearned, so the body can unwind. As this happens, both physical and emotional restrictions are released. This is myofascial unwinding.

This process of unwinding and change has been described as removing layers, like peeling an onion. As each layer is uncovered, or rather re-discovered, people feel a regression through the stages of their symptoms, until they reach the original pain that started it all. They are often surprised by the familiarity with which they can greet their old pain and then let it go.

Many people are taken aback by the power of what is a very gentle and slow therapy. They sometimes relive memories and experience involuntary twitches, physical movements, and emotions as the fascia releases. Rather than being disturbing, these are experienced positively as a letting go.

Often the work is deeply relaxing, although accompanied by "good" pain. The releases people experience during a myofascial release therapy session are only the start of the process, and many people find their body and mind continue to unwind and release for many days and weeks afterwards.

Sometimes a person can go through a physical unwinding process in which movement is progressively restored, but without feeling any pain relief. This person is focused on their pain to such an extent that their mind–body responds to the physical unwinding by continuing to push itself to the limit of pain. It is only when the "new normal" is pointed out to them that they consciously realize what has been happening and start to feel pain relief.

The unwinding process can give rise to a range of emotions and can sometimes feel like a roller coaster of change. This is perfectly normal and the change and movement are good. They are signs that your mind–body is paying attention to the therapy and that balance is returning.

The irony of any chronic pain is that it takes the body a massive amount of energy to maintain the physical restrictions that cause the pain, and an equally massive amount of mind energy to maintain the awareness of pain. One of the common early effects of myofascial release is a sense of increased physical energy and mental lightness as the tissue releases cause the release of stuck energy. Even when a painful layer is shed you are progressing towards a more positive future.

What this means for helping yourself

The same understanding and qualities that make myofascial release an effective hands-on therapy can be used and adapted to create effective self-help techniques. With an appreciation of the fascial body, and the processes by which pain is felt, it is possible to release fascial restrictions within your own body, and to rebalance physically and emotionally.

A knowledge of the unwinding process, and what it is possible to achieve, can help to sustain you through a process of change, or as you enlist the help of supportive friends and family.

With a little practice and patience, you can learn to work positively with your fascia and experience your own unwinding, knowing that your mind–body will release only what is holding you back.

Just remember:

- your fascia is a three-dimensional web providing support throughout your body
- your fascia naturally wants to stay balanced and move freely
- gentle sustained pressure creates the space for your fascia to unwind, returning you to your natural pain-free you.

Help Yourself Out of Chronic Pain

Life is the sum of all your choices.

Albert Camus

In this chapter we explore:

- using what you now know about fascia
- taking a holistic approach to helping yourself out of chronic pain
- ways to improve your fascial health and therefore your whole health.

Life events combine to create fascial restrictions that can lead to chronic pain conditions. We each have a unique combination of life experiences, physical injuries and changes, emotional responses and habits. These all come together to create our mental and physical selves.

Narrow medical approaches, such as medication and surgery, often do not work for chronic pain conditions. Sometimes they can make matters worse. And often we are told we will just have to live with it. It is therefore up to us to find more holistic solutions to help ourselves.

You get to choose

I chose to specialize as a myofascial release therapist because, of all the hands-on therapies I sampled and trained in, myofascial work made the most sense and got the best results. Over many years of treating clients my belief in a holistic myofascial approach to chronic pain has been rewarded again and again as clients who had given up hope or been abandoned by the medical profession have got well again and been able to live pain-free lives. Aside from the hands-on work itself, what my clients have most valued are:

- an explanation about how chronic pain happens
- simple ways to help themselves.

My intention in writing this book is to share more widely the information and self-help techniques that have most helped my clients.

Knowledge is power. Having read as far as here, you already have much more knowledge about the fascinating world of fascia and about how your mind–body really works. You are no longer a passive patient waiting for things to be done to you. You are an empowered individual who can make positive changes that will make a difference to your life from now on.

In this book I have emphasized the fact that you are unique and individual and therefore that the pain you currently feel is as unique as you are. Your path to recovery is also unique and is yours to take.

The uniqueness of each person's journey is the reason I have not created a one-size-fits-all plan for you to follow. In keeping with this basic holistic principle, I have considered many different aspects of recovery and I am setting before you different options so you can make informed and positive choices and take with you what feels right. In this way you will give your mind–body the best opportunity to recover its balance and to free yourself from pain, for good. As an empowered individual, the choices are all yours.

On your path to recovery, you may discover other pieces of the recovery puzzle and approaches that resonate and make sense to you, and which are not covered in this book. If they feel right, then they probably are right for you – remember that fascial gut feeling!

Using what you know about fascia

Fascia is everywhere within your body; it is the connecting connective tissue. Everything you do, every movement you make (or do not make), every thought you have, all affect your fascia.

Knowing this, you can choose to become more fascially aware. I am not suggesting you read endless articles and books about fascia, just that you take the time to tune in to your fascia and notice how happy and healthy it feels. As you do, remember (from Chapter 5) that the very act of observing your fascia, of paying attention to it, will change the ways in which it behaves. So by becoming more fascially aware you are already creating changes that will benefit your body.

When you are still

When you have been still for a while, maybe sitting at your desk, close your eyes so you can focus on yourself, and notice where things might just be feeling a little tight, or perhaps a bit niggly. You might notice that you feel a bit of pain there, or maybe just a sensation of things being not quite right. This is a fascial restriction starting to form.

So, imagining the fluid nature of fascia, try moving that part of your body, even just very slightly. Notice what happens. Notice how the sensation shifts and releases.

When you move

Choose any movement you like, maybe reaching out for the kettle, or up to a cupboard. Whatever speed you are moving at, slow it right down. Imagine all the strands of that movement stretching, adapting, and spreading through the fascial web, making connections, and releasing energy as your extracellular fluid flows.

As you stretch as far as you can comfortably go, notice the subtle sensations of tingling and warmth that mean your fascia is releasing and letting go.

When you think

Feelings of anxiety and calm come and go throughout each day, but it may not be until after these moments have passed that you become aware of how they have affected you. You know now that emotional reactions happen unconsciously and that they affect your fascia. The more aware you become of your patterns of reaction, the easier it becomes to change your emotions so they become more fascia friendly.

Fascial thinking

Try this simple mind exercise to tune into your fascial patterns of emotion. (You might like to record these words so that you can experience the full effect without interruption):

Sitting calmly for a few minutes, just focus on your breathing and allow it to slow and become calm and relaxed. Feel the breath moving in and out through your nose or mouth. Notice how your body feels – your rate of breathing, your heart rate, your arms and legs – relaxed, slow, calm.

Now imagine a peaceful scene – it may be lying on a beach in the sun, it may be walking through some woods. Whatever comes to mind for you is just fine. Allow yourself a few minutes to think of this scene and ask your mind to make this as real as possible for you – maybe you can imagine yourself being there, seeing the colors, hearing the sound of the waves or your feet crunching through the leaves.

Now tune in again to how your body is feeling – your rate of breathing, your heart rate, your arms and legs – and notice how everything feels.

How much more calm and relaxed do you feel now? What emotions come to mind?

Now imagine another scene, a recent event when you felt anxious or stressed – maybe something happened at your work, or you had an argument with someone. Whatever comes to mind is just fine. Allow yourself to think of this scene and ask your mind to make this as real as possible – imagine yourself in the moment, how you felt, what you said.

Now tune in again to how your body is feeling – your rate of breathing, your heart rate, your arms and legs – and notice how everything feels.

Where do you feel tension now? What other sensations can you feel in your body? What emotions come to mind?

Before you finish, allow yourself a few moments of calm and steady breathing so your body can relax once more.

This simple exercise helps you to notice the power of your emotions and the effect they have on your fascia. Anxiety and stress can create fascial tension, often in areas you might not have imagined. Sometimes these emotions are enough to trigger familiar chronic pain symptoms.

Likewise, calming and relaxing emotions, such as joy and pleasure, allow your fascia to relax and let go. It really is as simple as that.

You can practice imagining your relaxing scene as often as you like. Each time you do it will help your fascia to develop new positive relaxed habits. And then next time you are feeling stressed or anxious, you have a new tool to help your fascia release those negative emotions.

Introducing the slow fix

We already know that everything in the mind–body interconnects with everything else. We know we have an intricate and multi-layered self-regulating fascial feedback system. And this system can be significantly affected by our emotions, as you will have experienced in the last exercise.

If you believe that you can heal yourself and remove pain, your body will respond by speeding up the healing response and reducing feelings of pain. If you believe that you are stuck with your pain and cannot heal, then your body will again respond accordingly.

Understanding this self-regulating placebo and nocebo system is vital in returning your mind–body to balance. The more you truly believe that you can recover, the more you will recover.

In this process it is important to understand that there is no quick fix to chronic pain. This may come as a disappointment to some people, but it is a fact. Too often, too many people become over-reliant on the medical profession, hoping that a new pill or a new procedure will be the instant miracle cure. Many non-medical approaches also promote this quick-fix mentality and people can hop from one approach to another in the hope that this will be the quick cure they are searching for.

However, the physical and mental reality is that you need to take the long-term view when it comes to controlling your own health. Moving to a pain-free life is about addressing balance in and between all aspects of your life, not just one or two. In this way you ensure that positive changes are nourished and become new and powerful mental, physical, and emotional habits. Understanding that you have the power within you to do and change whatever you want in your mind–body, the change you want can be as simple as deciding to change.

The cells in your body are built to replace and renew themselves. It takes around 6 months of regular bodywork to change your fascia. In this time you can remove excess stuck collagen, restore flexibility to your elastin, and return fluidity to your tissues. Just as your body has gradually become stuck, so it can gradually become unstuck. You can work with your body to help release your fascia through regular healthy stretching and movement activities. This is the principle of slow fix.

Applying the principle of slow fix to your mind–body means you can embrace a multi-tasking approach to change. Just as everyone is unique, the combination of techniques that will work for you will also be unique.

Chapter 11 contains a collection of effective self-help activities, stretches, and exercises. These are ones I use every day and pass on to my clients. They are all simple things that virtually anyone can do and which my clients find particularly helpful.

But first, let us start with some basic principles of holistic good health. It is likely that you have heard some of these suggestions before, and this is your opportunity to consider them again from a fascial perspective. Knowing what you now know about fascia and how you can positively improve your fascial health, you might just start to look at these ideas a bit differently and figure out where they fit in your holistic jigsaw of a healthy pain-free life.

Fascia-friendly breathing

When we talk about breath, we are really talking about the importance of correct breathing for our health. Much has been written about correct breathing over the years, particularly about mindful breathing and meditation. However, to emphasize the relationship between breath and fascia I am going to call it fascial breathing here. I am also going to go beyond the usual general assurances that deep breathing is good for you, to actually explain how and why it is such a powerful technique.

Breathing is essential for life. It is part of our two basic states of being: rest and digest and fight or flight (Chapter 7). As we have already seen, when we are in chronic pain and stressed, we spend too much of our time in fight or flight response. In fight or flight we alter how we breathe. Fight or flight breathing is shallow, it is mostly in the top of our ribcage, and it involves using some of the muscles in our neck to assist. Although helpful in fight or flight situations, prolonged shallow breathing like this increases our stress levels and promotes chronic respiratory conditions such as asthma.

From a fascial perspective, shallow breathing contributes to a tightening of the tissues in our neck, shoulders, and upper chest. The body struggles to deliver enough oxygen to the rest of the body and to remove carbon dioxide, the waste product of breathing. As a result, our fascia can become progressively more toxic and stuck, which leads to more restriction and pain.

Fascial breathing helps to counteract this. Fascial breathing engages the rest and digest part of our nervous system. By practicing fascial breathing on a regular basis, you are helping to retrain your mind and body into a calmer and more relaxed way of being. All of which benefits your fascial health both in the short and the longer term.

Fascial breathing promotes, amongst other things, a change in your brain waves. Through fascial breathing we can attain a relaxed "twilight" state of mind, where you are half-awake, half-asleep (sometimes described as "mind awake, body asleep"). In this state you are allowing your body to rest, relax, and repair.

Fascial breathing also promotes a healthy vagus nerve (Chapter 6). We talked about it before in relation to whole mind and body health. The vagus nerve is unique in that it wanders throughout the body, enervating the throat, lungs, heart, and digestive system. It also connects with other nerves linked to social interaction such as eye contact, speech, recognition and understanding of facial expressions, voices, and so on.

The health of the vagus nerve is called vagal tone. When you have high vagal tone you have a healthy vagus nerve. This increases your ability to cope with stress, and improves your immune system, social interaction, and empathy. It also has a positive effect on memory and concentration. Low vagal tone, on the other hand, typically results in low mood, depression, and chronic inflammation, leading to chronic disease such as diabetes and heart attack and a low level of social interaction.

As far back as 1921, research by Otto Lowi demonstrated that by stimulating the vagus nerve we can decrease our heart rate and stimulate the release of a particular neurotransmitter that enables us to calm down.

There are many ways in which you can help to improve the health of your vagus nerve, such as exercise and learning new things, but one of the most powerful is through fascial breathing. When you breathe fascially, your body simply cannot stay in fight and flight, and it has to move into rest and digest mode. This plays an important part in relaxing your fascia and helping your body out of chronic pain.

As you practice fascial breathing regularly you will soon notice the benefits. Most importantly, you will have a powerful tool for any stressful situation in the future. For example, if you find yourself stressed at work or sitting an exam, a few minutes fascial breathing beforehand will calm your nervous system, focus your mind, and put you in a strong position for the task ahead.

How to breathe fascially

First make sure that you are in a relaxed, quiet space and make yourself comfortable, whether seated or lying down. Tune into your breath and notice where and how you are breathing. Are you breathing through your nose, your mouth, or both? Is your ribcage moving as you breathe, or does your breath feel tight and shallow?

When you first start to practice fascial breathing, it is a good idea to place the palms of your hands on your lower ribs. This way you can notice how your ribcage moves when you breathe. If your diaphragm is engaged, then your ribs will move out and slightly up towards your head as you breathe in, and then in and slightly down towards your feet as you breathe out. It is a good idea to practice this a few times before you start so you get the feeling in your hands and your body. The aim of fascial breathing is to move your lower ribcage by breathing with your diaphragm.

Then start to breathe in a pattern of 7/11 breathing – breathe in for a count of 7 and out for a count of 11. When you finish breathing out, just allow yourself to be still for a moment before breathing in again. This still point encourages further deep relaxation in the body.

If you find that you are struggling towards the end of either the in-breath or the out-breath, or if you feel you have to force the end of your out-breath, then simply adjust the count for both until you feel comfortable. Always keep the out-breath longer than the in-breath, as this helps to stimulate the rest and digest system. The most important thing is that you feel comfortable and relaxed throughout, not forcing or rushing anything – just noticing your breaths and the pauses in between.

At first just practice fascial breathing for 5 minutes a day. As your body gets used to it, you can then adjust the count for the in-breath and the out-breath, if necessary, until you can comfortably manage the 7/11 count. Gradually increase the time you spend practicing until you can manage 10 to 15 minutes. This is something that you can combine with the towel stretch (see Chapter 11) for maximum relaxation benefit.

Fascia-friendly nutrition

This is not a book about nutrition, and I am not about to give you a healthy eating plan. Instead, I am just going to mention some key points about how what you eat and drink affects your fascia. As we already know, fascia is made of protein and water. How these come to be in our body in the first place is through what we eat and drink.

Water, water everywhere ...!

A lot has been written about water – maybe too much. And the official advice has changed over time so we can all be forgiven for being confused, unsure about when and how much to drink. While it is possible to drink too much water in certain circumstances, virtually every single one of us drinks too little water.

From a fascial perspective, if you are in chronic pain your fascia is stuck. If your fascia is stuck, it is dehydrated. And if your fascia is dehydrated, then your whole body is dehydrated. It only takes a 2% drop in body fluid levels to affect the performance of all our body systems. Most people in chronic pain are also chronically dehydrated.

The relationship between stuck fascia and dehydration is a vicious circle. Sometimes dehydration starts it; the fascia is dehydrated so it becomes viscous and sticky, and then stuck. Sometimes an injury occurs, which literally squeezes the water out of the fascia, a bit like squeezing a bath sponge tight, resulting in further restrictions, and so it goes on.

If you want to help rehydrate your fascia, in tandem with your self-help activities, stretches, and exercises, then you should drink 1.5 to 2 liters of water a day. Water is the important fluid here. Anything containing caffeine, such as coffee or tea, is a diuretic and will only dehydrate you further, as will alcohol. Anything containing refined sugar, such as soft drinks and sodas, can also dehydrate your tissues. Diet drinks are no better as the sugar has been replaced by chemicals which are actually toxic to the body and can cause health issues.

So water is really important. You get to choose tap water, bottled water, filtered water, still or sparkling! You can pep it up with some fresh squeezed lime or lemon. You can also choose to substitute some of your water with herbal teas. The choice is yours.

If you do not believe me, try it for 10 days in combination with releasing your fascia. You may pee a lot at first, but this is because your dehydrated tissues cannot absorb all of the water you are putting into your body. However, as you stretch and release your fascia more, gradually your tissues will retain more of the fluid. As they do, you will start to feel better. You will feel less tired, and more energized. Your body will work more efficiently to detoxify itself and it will start to feel like it is moving well, more fluidly.

Eating for your fascia

Like every other part of our body, fascia needs healthy nutrition to help it repair itself and grow. Proteins are the building blocks of fascia, but energy in the form of carbohydrates and minerals are also needed to power the body processes that engage fascia. If we do not get this from a healthy diet then we do not get it at all.

To support your fascial health, the UK National Health Service (NHS) guidelines for healthy eating are a good place to start:

Base your meals on starchy carbohydrates

In themselves, starchy carbohydrates such as potatoes, bread, rice, pasta, and cereals are not fattening; it is the things we add to them that add fat. Choose wholegrains and potatoes with their skins on as they contain more fiber. Starchy carbs should make up one-third of your meals.

Eat lots of fruit and vegetables

Five a day is the guideline, but the more the better when it comes to fruit and veg, remembering to eat them in a healthy manner – not covered in cream or butter!

Eat oily fish

Fish is a great source of protein and contains many vitamins and minerals essential to the functioning of fascia.

Cut down on saturated fat, processed sugars, and salt

Saturated fats clog up our arteries, processed sugar is a toxin, and salt can raise blood pressure. All are best consumed in moderation as an excess will have an effect on fascial health. Most things that come in a packet will contain some fat, processed sugar, and salt, even when you might not expect it.

As a rule, keep your diet as close to nature as possible. Where possible make your meals from scratch. Remember that anything in a packet has been processed in some way, so limit the amount of packaged foods you eat.

The foundations of fascial health

The suggestions in this chapter all link back to what we already know about fascial anatomy. They are all suggestions for improving general fascial health and they will all work.

Now let us move on to consider more specific self-help techniques for particular areas of the body and chronic pain conditions.

Typical Chronic Pain Conditions

The burden of musculoskeletal disorders is huge – each year 20% of the
general population consult a GP about a musculoskeletal disorder.
Professor John Newton, Chief Knowledge Officer,
Public Health England

Introduction to the chronic pain conditions

The majority of chronic pain conditions are caused by musculoskeletal disorders,
that is, situations where fascial restrictions are causing imbalance and malfunction
in muscles, bones, and associated tendons and ligaments. Diagnoses may be given
by a general practitioner, a specialist, or many people end up self-diagnosing.

This chapter contains a selective list of many of the diagnoses people come to me
with. I treat many more people who have no diagnosis but have pain in particular
body areas. This list is organized by body area and then typical diagnosed chronic
pain condition. So you can search by body area or by diagnosed condition, or you
can just read through.

I have already said I am somewhat skeptical about some medical diagnoses of
chronic pain conditions (see Chapter 2). Just because you have a pain in a particular
area does not mean that you have a particular condition. However, a diagnosis can
be a useful starting point.

The following list refers first to a body area and then to a commonly diagnosed
condition affecting that area. Under each listed condition I have summarized
key points about the medical understanding of the condition and a fascial
understanding of the condition. All of the suggested self-help activities, stretches,

and myofascial ball work exercises listed under each condition are described in detail in Chapter 11. These suggestions are starting points. If you like the look of another exercise or find it helpful there is nothing to stop you doing that one as well – but more of that in Chapter 11.

Remember that just because a pain is felt in one part of the body does not mean that the originating problem is located there (Chapter 6). The self-help activities, stretches, and myofascial ball work exercises given in this book all relate to where the problem is most likely to have originated rather than to where the pain may be felt.

Head and neck: headaches, migraines, and new daily persistent headache (NDPH)

Typical symptoms

Headaches and migraines affect people in different ways. The distinction between the two is generally that a headache presents with head pain as the predominant symptom, whereas migraine symptoms may include nausea, vomiting, sensitivity to light and sounds, visual changes, vertigo, or, in the case of silent migraines, no actual pain.

The pain of headaches can also take many forms including throbbing, sharp pain, pressure, stabbing pain through the eye, and dull background ache.

Medical approaches

Medical approaches usually focus on medication to mask or reduce the symptoms.

Fascial understanding

Both headaches and migraines can be caused or exacerbated by restrictions in the fascia of the neck, shoulders and head. In many cases, the fascial restrictions cause abnormal tension in the muscles in these areas, especially the neck and shoulder muscles that attach into the bones of the skull. Sometimes the main restrictions are held more deeply in the meninges, which are the fascial layers surrounding the brain and spinal cord.

Fascial activities

The recommended fascial activities are designed to relax the whole mind–body and therefore to relieve tension in both the fascia and the nervous system. You may wonder why fascial squatting is recommended for headaches and migraines, but in my experience many people who have these conditions also have restrictions in their pelvis that contribute to their symptoms.

Fascial stretches

The recommended fascial stretching exercises focus on stretching the back as well as the neck and shoulders. I have also included a stretch for the front of the throat because many people who have headaches and migraines also suffer from tension in their face and jaw, which contributes to their symptoms.

Myofascial ball work

The recommended exercises focus on releasing tension in the neck, which is a primary source of pain, as well as in the back, which can also hold tension that travels up into the neck and head.

General fascial activities	Fascial stretches	Myofascial ball work
Any	S1, S2, S3	B1, B2, B3

Fascial stretches and myofascial ball work: slowly, gently and for at least 90 to 120 seconds for each one.

Head and neck: neck pain, torticollis, whiplash

Typical symptoms

To state the obvious, neck pain, as distinct from headaches, is pain felt in the neck itself. However, this pain is often accompanied by a stiffness in movement or a restriction in the range of movement, in particular turning the head from side to side.

Neck pain is often described as a nagging pain or even as a desire to stretch and release the restrictions that cause the pain. Sometimes people also develop crepitus, which is the crunchy sound you may experience as you turn your neck, caused by tightness in the fascia and muscles.

Torticollis is another name for wry neck, which is when you crick your neck and end up holding it at a painful angle.

Whiplash is injury to the soft tissues in the neck typically caused by a sudden deceleration, as in a car crash. However, many people can give themselves a whiplash injury by, for example, stepping off a higher than expected kerb and jarring their body, the jolt from which travels all the way from their foot to their neck.

Medical approaches

Medical approaches to neck pain are usually medication, heat, neck collars, and possibly physiotherapy.

Fascial understanding

Neck pain occurs when the fascia and muscles in the neck and shoulders become restricted. Apart from whiplash, an obvious cause is prolonged computer use when the fascia tightens to hold the weight of the head in a forward position. This causes the muscles to become tight and weakened, and irritates the nerves in the area. Whiplash can sit in the body for many years before developing into pain and is often linked to an imbalance in the pelvis.

Fascial activities

The recommended fascial activities are designed to relax the whole mind–body and therefore to relieve tension in both the fascia and the nervous system. Fascial squatting is included to help relax and rebalance the pelvis.

Fascial stretches

The recommended fascial stretches focus on stretching the back as well as the neck and shoulders. I have also included a stretch for the front of the throat because many people who have neck pain also suffer from tension in their face and jaw which contributes to their symptoms.

Myofascial ball work

The recommended exercises focus on releasing tension in the neck and shoulders, which is a primary source of pain, as well as in the back, which can also hold tension that travels up into the neck and head.

General fascial activities	Fascial stretches	Myofascial ball work
Any	S1, S2, S3	B1, B2, B3

Fascial stretches and myofascial ball work: slowly, gently and for at least 90 to 120 seconds for each one.

Head and neck: tinnitus

Typical symptoms

Tinnitus is noise in the ears which people variously describe as ringing, buzzing, humming, grinding, whistling, or whooshing. It is often worse at night or when there are fewer external noises to distract you. For some people it is position-related, that is, it is worse when the head or neck is in a particular position. For other people it is tension-related, and they can change their symptoms by clenching or relaxing their jaw.

Medical approaches

Medical approaches to tinnitus include ear irrigation to remove any excess ear wax, cognitive behavioral therapy (CBT) or counseling to help manage the symptoms, and using other sounds (such as music) to mask the tinnitus and help with sleep.

Fascial understanding

In the absence of any underlying issue such as hearing loss, tinnitus is commonly caused by restrictions in the fascia and muscles of the neck, shoulders, and head. The fascial lines in this area and the attachment points for muscles all converge on the base of the skull and the bones external to the ear. As with all things fascial, other areas of the body can also contribute, such as restrictions in the back and pelvis.

Fascial activities

The recommended activities are designed to relax the whole mind–body and therefore to relieve tension in both the fascia and the nervous system. Fascial squatting is included to help relax and rebalance the pelvis.

Fascial stretches

The recommended fascial stretching exercises focus on stretching the back as well as the neck and shoulders. I have also included a stretch for the front of the throat and the chest because tension here can contribute to additional pressure on the tissues leading into the ears.

Myofascial ball work

The recommended exercises focus on releasing tension in the neck and shoulders, which are primary sources of pain, as well as in the back, which can also hold tension that travels up into the neck and head.

General fascial activities	Fascial stretches	Myofascial ball work
Any	S1, S2, S3	B1, B2, B3

Fascial stretches and myofascial ball work: slowly, gently and for at least 90 to 120 seconds for each one.

Head and neck: temporomandibular joint (TMJ) and jaw pain

Typical symptoms

TMJ and jaw pain can be intense. The pain can be felt in the temporomandibular (jaw) joint itself, as well as in the teeth, face, ears, neck, and head. In addition to pain, people often also experience popping and clicking noises when they move their jaw, difficulty with eating and with opening and closing their mouth.

TMJ issues are often caused by stress and resulting bruxism (see below), but can also happen following dental procedures where the mouth is held open for prolonged periods.

Medical approaches

Dental treatment of TMJ can include a night splint, which can actually worsen the problem because it changes the tensions in the way your jaw is held.

Medical approaches include medication, cortisone injections, wearing a night splint, relaxation and, in some cases, surgery to address any dysfunction of the joint.

Fascial understanding

TMJ and jaw pain are caused by restrictions in the fascial mechanism of the jaw, in particular restricting the muscles of chewing. As these tissues tighten, they can cause the jaw to move out of alignment, also causing pressure on the discs in the TMJ joints. Restrictions in the jaw mean that your teeth are pushed together and this can result in tooth clenching or grinding (bruxism), especially at night. Sometimes dental work or wearing a night splint can alter the natural bite and this can also create fascial restrictions. However, the single biggest cause of TMJ is stress, which can cause people to unconsciously and repeatedly clench their jaw until the fascia gets stuck.

Fascial activities

The recommended fascial activities are designed to relax the whole mind–body and therefore to relieve tension in both the fascia and the nervous system. Fascial squatting is included to help relax and rebalance the pelvis, which is often pulled out of alignment by misalignment of the jaw.

Fascial stretches

The recommended exercises focus on stretching the back as well as the neck and shoulders. I have also included a stretch for the front of the throat and the chest because tension here can contribute to additional pressure on the tissues leading into the jaw.

Myofascial ball work

The recommended exercises focus on releasing tension in the neck, which is a primary source of pain, as well as in the back, which can also hold tension that travels up into the neck and head.

General fascial activities	Fascial stretches	Myofascial ball work
Any	S1, S2, S3	B1, B2, B3

Fascial stretches and myofascial ball work: slowly, gently and for at least 90 to 120 seconds for each one.

Repetitive strain injury (RSI): a word about RSI

Repetitive strain injury (RSI) is a controversial phrase. It is an umbrella term for various overuse injuries. Employers do not like the term because of its association with workplace practices that can give rise to legal liability and compensation claims. And medical doctors often do not like it because they prefer to narrow down the diagnosis to a more specific named condition.

Therefore, whether you are diagnosed with "RSI" depends on the approach of the doctor you see and the circumstances in which you are diagnosed. And whether you are diagnosed with one specific named overuse condition or another again depends on which doctor you see and the symptoms that are most predominant on that day.

In reality all RSI injuries are overuse injuries and may be caused by activities at work or outside work, and the symptoms may fluctuate daily to include the whole range listed under the various labeled conditions set out below. Therefore, when choosing your exercises, be guided more by where you are feeling restrictions and pain that day, rather than sticking rigidly to the exercises for only one named condition.

Neck, chest, and arms: RSI – thoracic outlet syndrome

Typical symptoms

The thoracic outlet is the space between your collarbone and first rib at the top of your chest. It is significant because the arm nerves (brachial plexus) and blood vessels pass through here on their way from the neck to the armpit. There are also some neck muscles which crowd the area further as they attach into the first and second ribs.

Thoracic outlet syndrome is compression of this area which causes symptoms typical of RSI including numbness, pain, and a sense of weakness anywhere from your shoulder down to your fingers. Sometimes the compression of blood vessels can also cause swelling and discoloration in the arm and hand.

Medical approaches

Medical approaches to thoracic outlet syndrome include medication, physiotherapy, and, in some cases, surgery to release the pressure by removing a portion of the first rib.

Fascial understanding

Thoracic outlet syndrome may be caused by a high-impact accident, such as a car accident, but it is most commonly the result of poor posture which develops from repeated computer use. This typically includes rounded shoulders and a forward head position which combine to compress the front of the chest. The fascial restrictions that result from poor posture and many hours seated in front of a computer screen, or looking down at a handheld device, hold the body in this stuck position.

Fascially, thoracic outlet syndrome is a limited diagnosis because the problem is never just in the thoracic outlet. Typically, anyone who has RSI symptoms has a whole chain of fascial stuckness from their head to their neck, shoulders, chest, back, arms, and hands.

Fascial activities

The recommended fascial activities are designed to relax the whole mind–body and therefore to relieve tension in both the fascia and the nervous system. The towel stretch is particularly good for opening out the chest and shoulders, releasing pressure on the thoracic outlet area.

Fascial stretches

The recommended exercises focus on stretching the neck, shoulders, and sides of the body, which can become restricted. I have also included a doorway stretch which helps to open out the front of the chest.

Myofascial ball work

The recommended exercises focus on releasing tension in the neck and shoulders, which are primary sources of pain, as well as in the back, which can also hold tension that travels down into the arms. I have also included an exercise to release the armpit because the brachial plexus (see above) continues its journey from the thoracic outlet down into the arm via your armpit. Often this area can become chronically tight as a result of holding your arms suspended for many hours while you type or use a mouse. There is also an exercise for releasing tightness in the hands that can help to start a sequence of releases back up to the chest.

General fascial activities	Fascial stretches	Myofascial ball work
Any	S1, S5, S6	B2, B4, B6

Fascial stretches and myofascial ball work: slowly, gently and for at least 90 to 120 seconds for each one.

Neck, chest, and arms: RSI – golfer's elbow and tennis elbow

Typical symptoms

Golfer's elbow and tennis elbow are also known by their medical terminology, medial epicondylitis and lateral epicondylitis. These refer to the tendinous attachments of the forearm muscles which typically become inflamed and painful in these conditions. It is possible to suffer from both conditions at the same time and to develop them without ever having touched a golf club or tennis racquet – in fact, only 5% of people develop these conditions from playing these sports.

Symptoms typically include pain on the inside or outside of the elbow, pain and weakness in the forearm, difficulty gripping things or turning your wrist – turning door knobs, for example.

Medical approaches

Medical approaches to golfer's elbow and tennis elbow include applying a brace just below the elbow to create a false attachment for the forearm muscles and to take the pressure off the elbow, and surgery to relieve the pressure in the area.

Fascial understanding

Golfer's elbow and tennis elbow are overuse injuries caused by excessive repetitive movements of the forearm muscles. These are groups of small muscles, packed tightly together into a small space. Their small size means they get tired easily and the repetitive movements of typing or carpentry, for example, mean they get irritated. This causes fascial changes which stick the muscles together into one irritated blob of tissue. The repetitive movement of the forearms also fatigues and irritates the arm nerves and their fascial sheaths, creating a line of fascial tension that extends from the neck to the fingers.

Fascial activities

The recommended fascial activities are designed to relax the whole mind–body and therefore to relieve tension in both the fascia and the nervous system. The towel stretch is particularly good for opening out the chest and shoulders, releasing the arm nerves, which can become compressed and irritated.

Fascial stretches

The recommended exercises focus on stretching the neck and arms to release tension in these areas. I have also included a doorway stretch to help release pressure on the thoracic outlet area.

Myofascial ball work

The recommended exercises focus on releasing tension in the neck, armpits, forearms, and hands, following the line of travel of the arm nerves. I do not recommend using a ball directly on the elbows themselves because (1) this will be incredibly painful and defeat the purpose of any intended release and (2) the elbows are only painful because the muscles and fascia attaching into them are over-tight – if you release the muscles and fascia the elbows will sort themselves out.

General fascial activities	Fascial stretches	Myofascial ball work
Any	S1, S4, S5	B2, B4, B5

Fascial stretches and myofascial ball work: slowly, gently and for at least 90 to 120 seconds for each one.

Neck, chest, and arms: RSI – carpal tunnel and tendonitis

Typical symptoms

The carpal tunnel is a narrow bony gap in the wrist through which the median nerve and tendons for the hand pass. Sometimes the tendons in this tunnel can become inflamed (called tendonitis), which puts pressure on the nerve. This causes symptoms such as pain, numbness, pins and needles, and loss of strength in the hand and fingers, and sometimes also the forearm.

Medical approaches

Carpal tunnel syndrome is diagnosed by a nerve conduction test in which sensors are placed above and below the carpal tunnel and an electrical current passed through. Loss of the signal means the median nerve is compromised. The medical approach is often to recommend surgery to relieve pressure. Other medical approaches include wearing a splint or having cortisone injections, or both.

Fascial understanding

Most diagnosed cases of carpal tunnel syndrome are nothing to do with the carpal tunnel. The symptoms are caused by fascial restrictions further "upstream," particularly in the neck, chest, and armpit, which are squeezing the arm nerves and causing the typical symptoms.

The symptoms typically start in the same way as all other RSI, through overuse of muscles that easily fatigue and become irritated. Computer work and manual work involving fine movements of the hands and wrists are the major causes.

Many people have needlessly undergone injections and surgery to the wrist, or had their wrists inconveniently immobilized by a splint when the source of the problem is not the wrist at all.

Fascial activities

The recommended fascial activities are designed to relax the whole mind–body and therefore to relieve tension in both the fascia and the nervous system. The towel stretch is particularly good for opening out the chest and shoulders, releasing the arm nerves, which can become compressed and irritated.

Fascial stretches

The recommended fascial stretches focus on stretching the neck and arms to release tension in these areas.

Myofascial ball work

The recommended exercises focus on releasing tension in the neck, arms, and hands, following the line of travel of the arm nerves.

General fascial activities	Fascial stretches	Myofascial ball work
Any	S1, S2, S4	B2, B5, B6

Fascial stretches and myofascial ball work: slowly, gently and for at least 90 to 120 seconds for each one.

Neck, chest, and arms: RSI – Dupuytren's contracture and trigger finger

Typical symptoms

Dupuytren's contracture and trigger finger are conditions affecting the fingers and thumb. In these conditions one or more fingers or the thumb can become stiff and difficult to move, in some cases getting stuck in a contracted claw-like position. Sometimes it is possible for someone to temporarily straighten their own finger or thumb (often accompanied by a popping noise) or sometimes it gets permanently stuck. Often an accompanying nodule develops in the palm of the hand at the base of the affected digit.

The condition is not usually painful but does affect movement.

Medical approaches

Medical treatment is usually surgery to release the tendon of the affected digit, but this is often unsuccessful long term as the condition can return.

Fascial understanding

Unsurprisingly, both of these conditions are caused by overuse of the arms and hands, which causes fascial thickening, in this case specifically in the palm of the hand and in the muscles and fascia of the forearms. As the forearms become more restricted, the tendons can no longer slide freely in the fascia to allow the fingers to bend and straighten. They become stickier and harder to move and eventually stuck. The nodules can develop as a form of scar tissue where the local fascia is repeatedly triggered to produce more and more collagen.

Fascial treatment of these conditions is similar to treating scar tissue: by breaking down the restrictions in the palm and forearms, the body is encouraged to reabsorb the excess tissue and return the forearm, hand, and fingers to normal movement.

Fascial activities

The recommended fascial activities are designed to relax the whole mind–body and therefore to relieve tension in both the fascia and the nervous system. The towel stretch is particularly good for opening out the chest and shoulders, releasing the arm and hand nerves, which can become compressed and irritated.

Fascial stretches

The recommended fascial stretches focus on stretching the neck and arms to release tension in these areas.

Myofascial ball work

The recommended exercises focus on releasing tension in the armpits, arms, and hands, which helps to break down the excess collagen formation.

General fascial activities	Fascial stretches	Myofascial ball work
Any	S1, S2, S4	B4, B5, B6

Fascial stretches and myofascial ball work: slowly, gently and for at least 90 to 120 seconds for each one.

Shoulders: rotator cuff injuries and frozen shoulder (adhesive capsulitis)

Typical symptoms

The shoulder is a shallow ball and socket joint held in place by muscles, ligaments and fascia, which means it allows a full rotational range of movement. The downside of this range of movement is that the shoulder can be quite susceptible to soft tissue injuries. The rotator cuff muscles allow this range of movement but are the most likely to become injured.

Rotator cuff symptoms can range from a dull ache and pain when sleeping on the affected side to restricted movement and sharp pain on certain movements because the tissues are impinged or pinched.

Frozen shoulder (adhesive capsulitis) is a condition in which the soft tissue capsule surrounding the shoulder joint becomes stuck together. This typically happens progressively over months or years and the shoulder can go through various stages from "freezing" to "frozen" and then "thawing" as it resolves.

At its worst frozen shoulder results in constant extreme pain, worse with movement, and very restricted movement in all directions. Frozen shoulder typically affects middle-aged women.

Medical approaches

Medically little is known about how frozen shoulder develops, and treatment can include surgery to decompress the joint. Other medical treatment for general shoulder conditions includes medication and cortisone injections.

Fascial understanding

Rotator cuff injuries can be caused by sports injuries, but most are due to overuse, whether through office or manual work. The same is true for frozen shoulder, but with the added element of stress which typically accumulates over many years before contributing to restricted movement conditions such as this, usually in middle age.

Frozen shoulder is often misdiagnosed when there is no adhesion in the shoulder joint at all. Instead the symptoms are caused by fascial restrictions in the supporting tissues surrounding the joint. Due to the normal high level of mobility of the shoulder, any restrictions can cause a high level of pain, even when it is not being used, purely due to the weight of the arm pulling on the restricted tissues.

The same goes for rotator cuff injuries and in both conditions, the muscles can literally become stuck together by the fascia leading to the restricted movement and pain that are common to both.

Fascial activities

The recommended fascial activities are designed to relax the whole mind–body and therefore to relieve tension in both the fascia and the nervous system. The towel stretch is not recommended for shoulder conditions as the gravitational pull of the stretch is often too painful to be tolerated comfortably. Fascial squatting is included to help relax and rebalance the pelvis, which is often pulled out of alignment by misalignment of the neck and shoulders.

Fascial stretches

The recommended fascial stretches focus on stretching the neck, back, and sides to release tension in these areas. At first you may need to adapt these depending on the amount of movement you have in your affected shoulder (see Chapter 11).

Myofascial ball work

The recommended exercises focus on releasing tension in the neck, back, and armpits, all of which become tight and restricted in these conditions. Care should be taken to position yourself comfortably as the pressure can sometimes be quite intense, especially around the armpit where rotator cuff restrictions are most likely to form.

General fascial activities	Fascial stretches	Myofascial ball work
Any	S1, S2, S6	B1, B3, B4

Fascial stretches and myofascial ball work: slowly, gently and for at least 90 to 120 seconds for each one.

Back and pelvis: upper, mid, or low back pain, prolapsed and bulging discs

Typical symptoms

The most commonly felt back pain is in the lower back, although pain can be felt anywhere from the neck down to the pelvis. Sometimes back pain is caused by other conditions, or a prolapsed or bulging disc, but in most cases there is no clear medical cause.

When discs bulge or prolapse they press on the nerves where the nerves exit from the spinal cord to travel to other parts of the body. Most typically this happens in the lower (lumbar) back because this is the main weight-bearing area. A prolapsed lumbar disc typically causes sciatica, which is a symptom not a condition, and sends pain, tingling, and numbness which can travel down through the buttock, groin, and leg to the foot. This type of sciatica is an unrelenting severe pain that affects sleep and all other day-to-day activities.

Other nonspecific back pain tends to cause a combination of pain felt in the back itself, and sometimes sciatica as well.

Medical approaches

Medical treatment of back pain is quite hands-off. The first approach is medication and physiotherapy exercises, and otherwise wait for 8 weeks as most disc problems resolve themselves within this time. Thereafter, if the pain continues, an MRI scan is required to see if it is a prolapse, in which case the usual solution is surgery.

Fascial understanding

Disc prolapses are interesting from a fascial perspective. Discs rarely prolapse spontaneously and a prolapse is usually the result of overuse, poor posture, and stress which leads to a tightening in the fascia and other tissues around the hips and back, to the point that the disc is squeezed out of place. It is like a jam doughnut being squashed to the point that the jam squirts out, the "jam" in this case being the centre of the disc, which then presses on the nerve, causing pain.

General back pain is the pre-prolapse stage, so anyone with back pain should take steps to get it resolved. Most lower back pain is actually caused by fascial and therefore muscle restrictions in the hips and groin; one of the major contributors is a muscle found in the front of the hip, the psoas, which is the main hip flexor (it allows you to lift your leg). Tightness in these tissues can squeeze the pelvic bones too tightly together, causing sacroiliac (SI) joint pain and pulling the whole structure out of balance so that the fascia and muscles in the back now have to take the strain without any help from the usual supporting tissues. In this sense back pain can be seen as an overuse problem.

Fascial activities

The recommended fascial activities are designed to relax the whole mind–body and therefore to relieve tension in both the fascia and the nervous system. Fascial squatting is included to help relax and rebalance the pelvis, which is always pulled out of alignment in back problems.

Fascial stretches

The recommended fascial stretches focus on stretching the back and hips to release tension in these areas. Spinal twist is also included to improve rotation in the lower back.

Myofascial ball work

The recommended exercises focus on releasing tension in the back, buttocks, and sides of the hips as tension in all of these areas contributes to pain felt in the back.

General fascial activities	Fascial stretches	Myofascial ball work
Any	S6, S7, S8	B3, B7, B8

Fascial stretches and myofascial ball work: slowly, gently and for at least 90 to 120 seconds for each one.

Back and pelvis: sciatica and piriformis syndrome

Typical symptoms

We have already encountered sciatica above. Sciatica is actually a symptom, although it is often given as a diagnosis. Piriformis syndrome can result in sciatica as well as pain directly in the buttock as the piriformis is a muscle found deep in the buttock. The piriformis is unique in that the sciatic nerve runs either through it or close to it in most people, so that tightness in the muscle squeezes the nerve.

Pain from this condition, and sciatica itself, can mimic a prolapsed disc.

Medical approaches

Medical approaches to sciatica and piriformis syndrome typically include medication, cortisone injections, physiotherapy, and, in rare cases, surgery to release pressure on the sciatic nerve.

Fascial understanding

Piriformis syndrome is caused by a tightening of the fascia in the buttocks, which squeezes the muscle and sciatic nerve. However, this is almost always accompanied by tightness in the fascia and other tissues all the way round the hips, creating a postural imbalance.

This condition is also known as "wallet syndrome," and is unique to men as it can be caused by the imbalance of habitually keeping a wallet in one of your back pockets. It is an underuse condition too, common in people who sit for a living – office workers and drivers, for example.

Fascial activities

The recommended fascial activities are designed to relax the whole of the mind–body and therefore to relieve tension in both the fascia and the nervous system. Fascial squatting is included to help relax and rebalance the pelvis which is always pulled out of alignment in back problems.

Fascial stretches

The recommended fascial stretches focus on stretching the back, hips, and legs to release tension in these areas. Spinal twist is also included to improve rotation in the lower back and relieve pressure on the buttocks.

Myofascial ball work

The recommended exercises focus on releasing tension in the buttocks, legs, and sides of the hips as tension in all of these areas contributes to pain felt in the buttocks.

General fascial activities	Fascial stretches	Myofascial ball work
Any	S7, S8, S10	B7, B8, B9

Fascial stretches and myofascial ball work: slowly, gently and for at least 90 to 120 seconds for each one.

Back and pelvis: chronic pelvic pain syndrome (CPPS), non-bacterial prostatitis

Typical symptoms

Chronic pelvic pain syndrome (CPPS) affects both men and women. Medically the causes for this condition are not really known. In women it is thought to be caused by endometriosis, fibroids, or irritable bowel syndrome, amongst other things. In men the causes are even more vague.

The symptoms of CPPS in both men and women are similar, and can include general pain in the pelvic region, both external and internal, pain on urination and defecation (and on ejaculation in men), genital pain, urinary frequency or problems with urination, general pains around the pelvis, groin, and lower back. Pain can vary from a dull ache to burning or sharp electric pains.

Non-bacterial prostatitis is a diagnosis given when men suffer from some or all of the above symptoms, which are also indicative of an infection of the prostate, but in this case no infection is present.

Medical approaches

In both conditions the medical approach is a bit scattergun. Men can be given repeated courses of antibiotics despite it being known there is no infection. Both men and women can be given painkillers, physiotherapy, and even psychotherapy.

Sometimes a consultant may perform a laparoscopy, in which a tube is inserted via an incision in the abdomen to look for possible causes (see scar tissue, below) and, in some cases, may perform a full or partial hysterectomy in women as a way of cutting out the problem. This often makes the problem worse not better.

Medically, both conditions tend to be regarded as incurable.

Fascial understanding

In my opinion, both CPPS and non-bacterial prostatitis are catch-all diagnoses for "we don't know what's going on there."

In women, there may well be endometriosis and/or fibroids present, but these are only part of the issue and may be caused by long-term fascial restrictions in the uterus.

The cause of CPPS and non-bacterial prostatitis is generally fascial restrictions externally around the hips, lower back, abdomen, and legs, and internally in the organs and pelvic floor. The abdominal and pelvic cavities lie one on top of another and both are tightly packed with organs and deep fascia. When coupled with a tight pelvic floor, the area becomes so restricted that the organs are literally squashed and they start to complain. The uterus and ovaries can become painful and produce abnormal tissues (for example, fibroids) and the prostate can no longer function properly.

Fascial restrictions in this area can be caused by too much sitting, too little stretching, and stress and anxiety, which is a major contributory factor in these conditions.

Fascial activities

The recommended fascial activities are designed to relax the whole mind–body and therefore to relieve tension in both the fascia and the nervous system. Fascial squatting is included to help relax and rebalance the pelvis, which is always pulled out of alignment in pelvic problems.

Fascial stretches

The recommended fascial stretches focus on stretching the sides and fronts of the hips to release tension in these areas. Spinal twist is also included to release the hips.

Myofascial ball work

The recommended exercises focus on releasing tension in the buttocks, legs, and sides of the hips as tension in all of these areas contributes to pain felt in the pelvis.

General fascial activities	Fascial stretches	Myofascial ball work
Any	S6, S7, S8	B7, B8, B9

Stretches and myofascial ball work: slowly, gently and for at least 90 to 120 seconds for each one.

Back and pelvis: chronic abdominal pain

Typical symptoms

Chronic abdominal pain can sometimes be linked to irritable bowel syndrome (IBS) or other digestive conditions but often there is no clear medical cause for it. It can often be an accompanying condition to chronic pelvic pain syndrome (CPPS).

The symptoms can include an underlying dull pain, episodes of sharp pain and cramps, diarrhea, constipation, bloating, and acid reflux. Stress generally makes the symptoms worse.

Medical approaches

Medical treatment usually involves a combination of pain-killing and antacid medications.

Fascial understanding

One of the main fascial causes of chronic abdominal pain is scar tissue from surgery and this is most commonly seen in women. Scars from Caesarian sections, hysterectomies, and the removal of endometriosis tissue and fibroids are the most common abdominal surgeries. Even performed by laparoscopy, or vaginally in the case of hysterectomies, the very act of removing something causes scar tissue to form.

The tension caused by the scar tissue often starts to create tightness in the hips and buttocks, as the scar tissue literally pulls everything closer together, and over time this can lead to other apparently unconnected pain conditions.

Very commonly the scar tissue will grow after surgery and over several years attach itself to other internal structures in the form of adhesions, at which point the pain starts to intensify. At this stage medical help may not be forthcoming. Women are often told that the original surgery was successful and that there is nothing to now complain about or they are told that the surgeon can "go back in" and cut out the scar tissue (causing yet more scar tissue).

Unsurprisingly, stress and anxiety caused by the pain and/or the attitude of the doctor often makes the condition much worse.

Fascial activities

The recommended fascial activities are designed to relax the whole mind–body and therefore to relieve tension in both the fascia and the nervous system. Fascial squatting is included to help relax and rebalance the pelvis, which is always pulled out of alignment in pelvic and abdominal problems.

Fascial stretches

The recommended fascial stretches focus on stretching the hips and legs to release tension that will have built up in these areas. A spinal twist is also included to release the hips.

Care should be taken with any exercises when there is abdominal scar tissue as it can be very sensitive to stretching, so be gentle and do little and often to build it up.

Myofascial ball work

The recommended exercises focus on releasing tension in the buttocks, legs, and sides of the hips as all of these areas can become tight.

General fascial activities	Fascial stretches	Myofascial ball work
Any	S6, S7, S8	B7, B8, B9

Fascial stretches and myofascial ball work: slowly, gently and for at least 90 to 120 seconds for each one.

Legs, hips, and feet: knee pain and runner's knee

Typical symptoms

Runner's knee is a catch-all term for general knee pain, also known as patellofemoral (patella = kneecap, femur = thigh bone) syndrome. Knee pain can be felt on the inside or outside of the knee, under the kneecap and sometimes even behind the knee. Pain can be sharp or a dull ache and can be linked to activities such as getting up from sitting, squatting, kneeling, going up or down stairs, or walking up or down hills. Sometimes it might also be accompanied by swelling and a popping or crunching sound (crepitus) when you move the knee.

Sometimes people can develop knee pain following surgery to repair a damaged ligament in the knee.

Medical approaches

Medical approaches to treating knee pain include icing the area, medication, cortisone injections, strapping the knee, physiotherapy to strengthen the quadriceps muscles, or orthotic inserts to change the way your foot supports you.

Fascial understanding

Many people are surprised to learn that one of the main fascial reasons for knee pain is an imbalance and facial restriction in the hips.

Your thigh bone is designed to rotate in your hip joint as you walk and run, it rotates out as you raise your leg and move it forward, and then back in as your foot plants onto the ground. This movement stabilizes your leg for weight bearing as it literally screws the top of the leg into the hip.

If you develop fascial restrictions in your hips from overuse, such as too much running, or underuse, such as too much sitting, then your leg will still try to rotate as you walk or run, but now, as well as being screwed into the hip, the force is transmitted down your leg to your knee. Meanwhile, fascial restrictions in your quadriceps (thigh muscles) can cause your kneecap, which sits in the tendon of your quadriceps, to slide to the left or right as you move. Finally, the changes in your gait are transmitted to your foot and can result in fallen arches as the weight now falls differently. The fascial structure in the arch of your foot is regarded as a vital structure from which your posture rises. Lose your foot arch and your whole posture can collapse.

Fascial activities

The recommended fascial activities are designed to relax the whole mind–body and therefore to relieve tension in both the fascia and the nervous system. Fascial squatting is included to help relax and rebalance the pelvis which is always pulled out of alignment in knee problems.

Fascial stretches

The recommended fascial stretches focus on stretching the hips, legs, and feet to release tension that will have built up in these areas.

Myofascial ball work

The recommended exercises focus on releasing tension in the buttocks, sides of the hips, and legs as all of these areas can become tight and affect your knees.

General fascial activities	Fascial stretches	Myofascial ball work
Any	S8, S9, S10	B7, B8, B9

Fascial stretches and myofascial ball work: slowly, gently and for at least 90 to 120 seconds for each one.

Legs, hips, and feet: shin splints

Typical symptoms

Shin splints are an overuse injury caused by running or walking too much, especially on hard surfaces, with poorly fitting shoes or by suddenly increasing activity levels. Symptoms include an aching pain in the shins which is directly related to weight-bearing exercise and can become sharp as it progresses.

Medical approaches

The medical approach is to rest, ice the area, and take painkillers and anti-inflammatories. The best "cure" for shin splints is to stop the activity that causes it.

Fascial understanding

Shin splints are most definitely an overuse problem, where the shin muscle is overworked. Because this muscle is fascially fixed to the shin bone down its entire length, when it becomes irritated, it irritates the bone too. This will cause fascial thickening as more collagen is produced and can lead to micro scars forming in the tissues.

Fascial activities

The recommended fascial activities are designed to relax the whole mind–body and therefore to relieve tension in both the fascia and the nervous system. Fascial squatting is included to help relax and rebalance the pelvis, which is always pulled out of alignment in any leg problems.

Fascial stretches

The recommended fascial stretches focus on stretching the hips, legs, and feet to release tension that will have built up in these areas.

Myofascial ball work

The recommended exercises focus on releasing tension in the hips and legs as these areas can become tight. I have also included working on the sole of your foot to help release the fascia and restore the arch to its proper shape, helping to release the shin muscle, which also attaches into the arch of the foot.

General fascial activities	Fascial stretches	Myofascial ball work
Any	S8, S9, S10	B8, B9, B10

Fascial stretches and myofascial ball work: slowly, gently and for at least 90 to 120 seconds for each one.

Legs, hips, and feet: chronic compartment syndrome and calf pain

Typical symptoms

Chronic compartment syndrome is a condition that affects the calf and causes a specific type of calf pain. In this condition, exercise causes an increase in blood flow to the calf, which is normal, but the fascia surrounding the muscles does not give to allow the muscles to swell.

Symptoms include aching, burning, or cramping pain, numbness, and weakness. All of the symptoms only come on with exercise and they stop again when you stop.

Other calf pain can be caused by minor damage to the tissues, often due to overuse.

Medical approaches

Medical approaches to this condition include recommended stretches and strengthening exercises, or surgery to cut into and even to remove the problem fascia.

Fascial understanding

The calf is a weight-bearing area of the body and also has a dual role of pumping fluids back up the body against gravity. Calf muscles are very powerful but constrained within tight fascial compartments. Overuse of the calves through weight training or running can cause facial restrictions to develop, and these impair the sliding ability of the tissue. Calf pain and chronic compartment syndrome can result from this tension.

Strengthening or cutting the fascia through surgery will only increase the problem.

Fascial activities

The recommended fascial activities are designed to relax the whole mind–body and therefore to relieve tension in both the fascia and the nervous system. Fascial squatting is included to help relax and rebalance the pelvis and knee and ankle joints, which can be a cause of calf problems.

Fascial stretches

The recommended fascial stretches focus on stretching the hips, legs, and feet to release tension that will have built up in these areas.

Myofascial ball work

The recommended exercises focus on releasing tension in the hips and the legs, as all of these areas will be tight. I have also included working on the sole of your foot as the tissue here is directly connected to the calf via the Achilles tendon so release here will help reduce tension in the calf.

General fascial activities	Fascial stretches	Myofascial ball work
Any	S8, S9, S10	B8, B9, B10

Fascial stretches and myofascial ball work: slowly, gently and for at least 90 to 120 seconds for each one.

Legs, hips, and feet: plantar fasciitis and heel spurs

Typical symptoms

Plantar fasciitis is the medical term for thickening and irritation of the fascia on the sole of the foot. This can cause heel pain and foot pain that is worse in the mornings or after sitting for a while. Walking can make it feel better although standing for long periods make it worse, hence its other name "policeman's heel."

Heels spurs are small protrusions of bone associated with plantar fasciitis. Sometimes the tension caused by the thickening fascia stimulates additional bone to grow along this line. Heel spurs can be painful when pressure is applied, as in walking or standing, but they are not always the source of pain.

Medical approaches

Medical approaches include rest, cortisone injections, night splints to stretch the sole of the foot, and orthotics. If these do not resolve the issue then plantar release surgery to cut the fascia away from the heel and remove heel spurs may be recommended.

Fascial understanding

The plantar fascia is a naturally thick layer of superficial fascia designed to protect the deeper structures of the foot. The superficial fascia on the sole of the foot (and that on the palm of the hand) is unique in that it does not slide. Imagine if it did – you would be sliding around all over the place and unable to hold things without dropping them.

Overuse of the feet, such as excessive standing, walking, or running, can cause the calf to tighten, as we have seen above. As this happens, the fascia in the calf tightens too and pulls on the Achilles tendon which attaches it to the heel. This line of tension continues round into the plantar fascia, pulling that tight too. The heel therefore becomes irritated and painful due to this extra pressure.

Fascial release of plantar fasciitis therefore focuses as much on the calf as on the foot.

Fascial activities

The recommended fascial activities are designed to relax the whole mind–body and therefore to relieve tension in both the fascia and the nervous system. Fascial squatting is included to help relax and rebalance the pelvis and knee and ankle joints, which can be a cause of calf and foot problems.

Fascial stretches

The recommended fascial stretches focus on stretching the hips, legs, and feet to release tension that will have built up in these areas.

Myofascial ball work

The recommended exercises focus on releasing tension in the hips and the legs as all of these areas will be tight. I have also included working on the sole of your foot to release tension here.

General fascial activities	Fascial stretches	Myofascial ball work
Any	S8, S9, S10	B8, B9, B10

Fascial stretches and myofascial ball work: slowly, gently and for at least 90 to 120 seconds for each one.

Pain syndromes: fibromyalgia, chronic fatigue syndrome (ME)

Typical symptoms

Fibromyalgia and chronic fatigue (or ME) are systemic conditions which can range across a spectrum of symptoms. Typically symptoms can include muscular and joint pain which moves around the body, extreme fatigue, brain fog, headaches, difficulty sleeping, depression, and digestive upsets. Depending on which symptoms predominate, a person can be diagnosed with either of these conditions.

Medical approaches

Medically these conditions are regarded as incurable and treatment includes ongoing medication, talk therapies such as cognitive behavioral therapy (CBT), and recommended lifestyle changes such as exercise and relaxation.

Fascial understanding

Both conditions are diagnosed based on the symptoms presenting on the day. In the case of fibromyalgia, people often have a tender point test, in which their doctor presses 18 specific points on the body. If at least 11 of these points are tender and the 11 are spread across both the upper and lower body on both sides, then fibromyalgia is diagnosed. However, many people receive a diagnosis with no specific test and without typical symptoms. In the worst example I have known, someone with limited pain in one upper arm, caused by overuse, was diagnosed with fibromyalgia by their general practitioner.

Fibromyalgia and chronic fatigue usually happen when a person's immune system, weakened by years of other pain conditions and general stress, can no longer cope. This triggers the unconscious nervous system into overdrive – often both the fight or flight and rest and digest systems are stuck full on, which is a bit like pressing the accelerator and the brake in a car at the same time.

Typically, these conditions develop following a major emotional event (such as the death of a loved one) or a viral infection, and typically they happen in middle age, just at the time when a person's years of multi-tasking, caring for others, builds to a crisis point. However, an increasing number of younger people (in their twenties and thirties) are also being diagnosed with these conditions.

Treating or self-treating fibromyalgia or chronic fatigue fascially requires care, as even the gentlest techniques can cause a disproportionately high response in an already overloaded system. Less is more, so take time to introduce techniques one at a time and allow time for the body to notice and adapt to the changes.

Fascial activities

The recommended fascial activities are gentle and designed to relax the whole mind–body and therefore to relieve tension in both the fascia and the nervous system.

Fascial stretches

The recommended fascial stretches focus on stretching the neck and include a spinal twist to help free the back.

Myofascial ball work

The recommended exercises focus on releasing tension in the back of the neck which will also help to release the vagus nerve (see Chapter 9) and therefore stimulate improved heart function, breathing, and digestion. I have also recommended using a ball on the hands and feet as a gentle way of releasing tension throughout the body without pressure on other pain-sensitive structures.

General fascial activities	Fascial stretches	Myofascial ball work
G4, G5	S1, S2, S7	B1, B6, B10

Fascial stretches and myofascial ball work: slowly, gently and for at least 90 to 120 seconds for each one.

Now time for some exercise

In the next chapter we describe how to do each of these activities, stretches, and exercises with options for beginners and for more advanced levels of fascial stretching. At the end of the chapter is a summary table of the exercises grouped by body area and diagnosed chronic pain condition.

Fascial Activities, Stretches, and Exercises

Any release is a good release.

John Barnes

In this chapter you will find:

- a selection of self-help activities, stretches, and myofascial exercises that will help you to get out and stay out of pain
- the activities, stretches, and exercises are all simple to do and can be adapted to suit your current pain level, flexibility, and mobility
- at the end is a summary of the activities, stretches, and exercises grouped by body area and diagnosed condition.

Introduction to the activities, stretches, and exercises

The main thing to remember when using any of these exercises is to stay within your comfort zone. Chronic pain symptoms can change from day to day, if not hour to hour, so it is always important to work with how you are feeling, not what you think you should do. If you are not feeling so great one day, then do things that are more relaxing for you.

There are three different types of activity and exercises for you to choose from:

- General fascial activities (G) – these are general fascial activities that are designed to help the whole body and can be done by most people.

- Fascial stretches (S) – these are fascial stretches that promote fascial release along tensional lines in the body. Fascial stretches can be done by most people but please read the section on when not to stretch (p. 178) before starting.
- Myofascial ball work (B) – these are exercises that require one or two myofascial release balls to promote fascial releases in specific areas of fascial tension and in muscle trigger points.

Some of these exercises may already be familiar to you, but it is unlikely that you will have done them fascially – and that's what makes the difference. Do them slowly, gently, and for at least 90 to 120 seconds each one, bringing to bear gentle pressure to release your fascia.

In the summary table at the end of the chapter I have grouped the activities, stretches, and exercises according to area of the body and diagnosed chronic pain conditions. This is just a convenient starting point. If you have a diagnosis you may be able to find it listed. If you just know it hurts somewhere you can start there. Once you are familiar with the exercises and the feel of fascial release, then you can start to explore some of the other stretches.

The general activities and fascial stretches do not require any special equipment. These are broad exercises designed to work on your whole body, or along mapped lines of fascial tension. The ball exercises require one or two myofascial release balls. These are small inflatable balls that come in a kit which is inexpensive to buy (Figure 11.1). Using the myofascial release ball kit enables you to do your own myofascial release, and helps you to work on hard-to-reach areas of the body. It is also portable, allowing you to use it at home, at work and even when travelling.

If your pain is caused by scar tissue, then any of these exercises will be helpful, again starting with the area where your scar is.

When you first start using these exercises it is a good idea to try

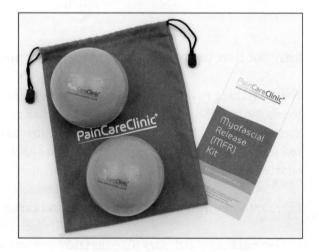

Figure 11.1: The Myofascial Release (MFR) Kit.

a short session of one type of exercise, say 10 minutes, then see how you feel the next day. Sometimes even the simplest of exercises can cause a temporary flare-up in your symptoms, especially if your fascia is very restricted. This is sometimes called a "healing crisis" and is a natural sign that something is shifting. If this happens, be kind to yourself. Wait until your fascia has settled and try something different. You can always come back to your first exercise again or find something that works better for you.

Once you are comfortable with 10 minutes you can build up the frequency and duration of your exercises. A good goal is 20 to 30 minutes a day. You can do this in one daily session or two or three shorter sessions during the day. You get to choose your own personal selection from any combination of the exercises we recommend. The main thing is to do whatever you do fascially – slowly and gently.

There are some people who choose to exercise for more than 30 minutes each day because they enjoy it. Some even carry their myofascial release ball kit around with them to use in spare moments. This may not be realistic if you have a busy lifestyle, and generally it is not necessary. However, it is good to do at least one thing to help yourself each day, even if it is only something small. The mental and emotional benefits of helping yourself each day can match the physical benefits. And anything you do will help to release the fascial restrictions that are causing your pain.

It is common sense that if an activity hurts, or makes the pain worse, then you should stop doing it.

Effect on your fascia

The exercises in this chapter are all a form of myofascial self-treatment. Whatever activity, stretch, or exercise work you are doing, the fascia throughout your body will respond and rebalance.

As everything is connected to everything else, even if an exercise directs you to work on one area, you may notice that your fascia starts to release in other areas and in different ways. This is the exciting thing about doing exercises fascially – every day and every stretch is different. Take your time to enjoy your fascial journey towards a pain-free you.

In releasing fascial restrictions you will also be releasing any trigger points (Chapter 6) that have formed. You can work directly on these using a ball and they will initially feel like intense areas of pain, but will then let go with a feeling of melting or relaxing of the tissues.

General fascial activities and how to do them

The general fascial activities are designed to help your whole body by supporting healthy unconscious physiological processes. Unless otherwise stated they can be done by everybody, and they can be done daily, even when you do not feel able to do anything else.

General activity 1 (G1): The towel stretch (not good for hypermobile people)

The towel stretch is a very simple exercise that can greatly help to relieve the poor posture that contributes to chronic pain.

Do the towel stretch because it:

- relaxes and stretches the girdles of the body, the shoulder and pelvic girdles
- helps to relax the nervous system.

Humans are bipeds. We have evolved to stand on two feet as opposed to all fours. This means that, unlike many animals which still have eyes on the sides of their heads and limbs on the sides of their bodies, humans have eyes positioned at the front and pointing forwards, and arms positioned and jointed for actions in front of us.

This focus to the front means that our posture has a tendency to slump forward, a factor that is further compounded by modern jobs and leisure habits. We may drive to work, sit in an office, face a computer screen all day, then sit to travel home, where we relax by again sitting on the sofa for what is left of the day.

Over time, our bodies respond to this pattern of use and our fascia starts to fix us in a forward position – very typically we develop a forward head position, we lose the natural curve in our necks, our shoulders become rounded and our pelvis tilts slightly forward (Figure 11.2).

It is these postural changes that often lead to the development of common chronic pain conditions such as lower back pain, RSI (repetitive strain injury), neck and shoulder pain, and so on.

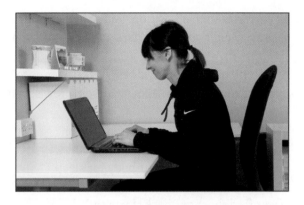

Figure 11.2: Typical poor computer posture – forward head position, flat back, rounded shoulders, and pelvis tilted forward.

How to use the towel stretch

Use a large towel like a bath sheet and roll it lengthways into a big sausage. If you do not have one towel that is long enough, you can place two rolled up towels end to end.

Place the towel on the floor and lie on it, face up, so that your spine is resting along the length of the towel.

Let your arms relax of the floor beside you and straighten your legs to lie flat on the floor (Figure 11.3).

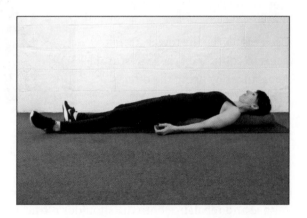

Figure 11.3: The towel stretch is a simple way of counteracting poor posture from computer use.

IMPORTANT – make sure that both your head and your bottom are on the towel. This is important because these are the areas where the rest and digest nerve fibres are clustered so that by lying on them you create a sustained pressure.

Read on below to find out why this is important.

Lie here for about 10–15 minutes and just let your body relax. It is best to set a timer so you can fully relax and, if you like, you can also listen to some relaxing music or a relaxation download. Maybe you can just do some fascial breathing, counting in for 7 and out for 11 (see below).

As you relax in this position, you will feel your body start to let go and gently stretch as gravity pulls your shoulders and pelvis down towards the floor.

At the end of the time, it is best to roll over onto your side and push yourself up into a sitting position. Allow yourself a few seconds for your body to readjust before getting up.

The towel stretch is a particularly good way of relaxing in the evening before bed as it will help to prepare your body for sleep.

If you find that your back starts to hurt or if you have any disc issues, you may find it more comfortable to bend your knees and place your feet on the floor (Figure 11.4).

Used regularly, the towel stretch helps to counteract these postural imbalances by using the effects of gravity to gently open out the restrictions at the front of the body and relax the back. The stretch helps to release tight chest muscles and creates more

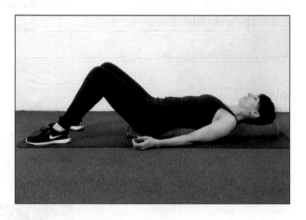

Figure 11.4: The towel stretch can be modified by bending your legs to alleviate lower back pain.

space for the arm nerves and blood vessels as they cross the chest. It also helps to release and rebalance both the shoulder girdle and the pelvic girdle, which are bony structures held in place by muscles, ligaments and fascia.

Used regularly, the towel stretch helps to engage the rest and digest system and restore balance to the body. It does this specifically by putting pressure on the base of the skull and on the sacrum at the base of the spine. In these areas are clustered the rest and digest nerve fibers which engage the digestive, respiratory, and cardiac systems, calming breathing and heart rate, relaxing muscles, and switching on the digestive and immune systems. This pressure also helps to release and improve the function of the vagus nerve, which is an essential part of the rest and digest response in the body.

Beginners – if the towel stretch is too strong, just lying on your back on the floor in the same position will have a similar beneficial effect (Figure 11.5).

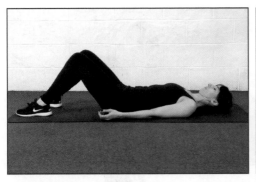 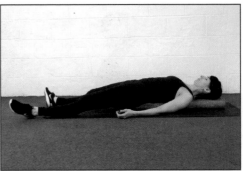

Figure 11.5: If the towel stretch feels too strong, just lie on your back on the floor.

Figure 11.6: For a deeper stretch, try using a foam roller.

Advanced – if you find this stretch is not enough, try using a foam roller (Figure 11.6) instead – you might want to wrap a towel round this first for comfort.

General activity 2 (G2): Spine roll-down (good for everyone)

You can do this as a part roll-down or a full roll-down, and either standing or seated. The principle is the same whichever you do. The main thing is to do it slowly and mindfully.

Prepare by thinking of your spine as a series of bones stacked one on top of the other. There are 24 moveable bones called vertebrae, running from the base of your skull down to your lower back just above your pelvis. Each should move independently of the others, but in many people the vertebrae have become stuck and can only move in groups. This stuckness leads to compressed or prolapsed discs, where the little shock absorber pads between each vertebra, are squeezed and eventually are pushed out of position.

Nerves extend from the spinal cord to all parts of the body. They exit the spinal cord through spaces between the vertebrae. These spaces can become compacted, which irritates the nerves. This exercise helps to widen these spaces, taking pressure off the nerves and preventing pain.

Starting at the top, tip your head forwards, and imagine your vertebrae slowly rolling forwards and down, one at a time. To ease the stretch, roll down each vertebra as you breathe out, and ensure that you do not allow your middle to slump – do this by

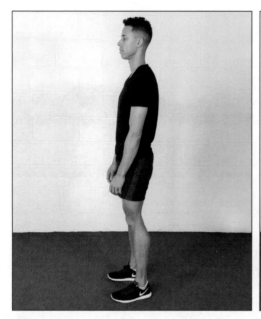

Figure 11.7: Spine roll-down start position with your head level and body relaxed.

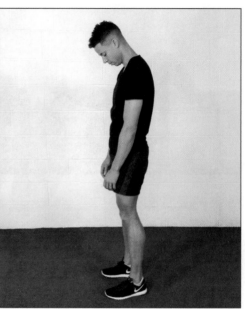

Figure 11.8: Starting at the top, tip your head forwards, and imagine your vertebrae slowly rolling forwards and down, one at a time, letting your arms hang loosely by your sides.

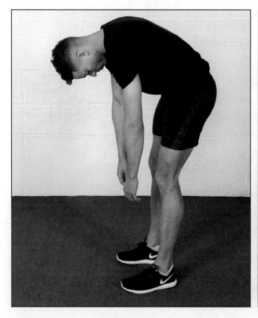

Figure 11.9: Part roll-down finish position – your hands should be somewhere below your knees.

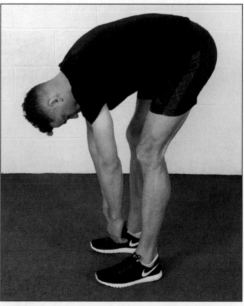

Figure 11.10: Full roll-down – your arms should be somewhere near the floor.

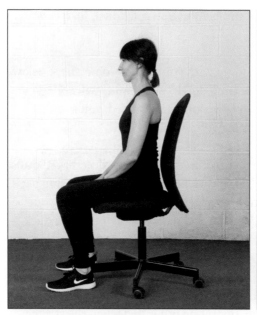

Figure 11.11: Seated spine roll-down start position – with your head level and legs spread to allow space for your body to roll down.

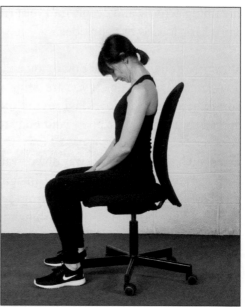

Figure 11.12: Seated roll-down – start by tipping your head forward and imagine your vertebrae rolling forward and down.

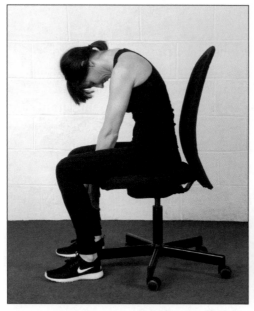

Figure 11.13: Seated part roll-down – finish position.

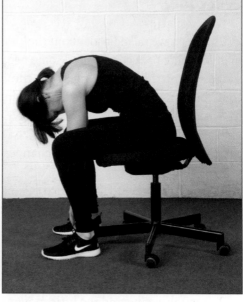

Figure 11.14: Seated full roll-down – finish position.

breathing actively and deeply into your ribs and belly as you roll down. Just let your arms hang loosely by your sides.

If you are doing a part roll-down, you will end up with your hands somewhere below your knees (Figure 11.9). If you are doing a full-roll down, your hands will end up somewhere near the floor (Figure 11.10). If you are doing this seated, you should spread your legs first to allow your body to roll right down.

Once you have rolled all the way down, wait there for a couple of slow deep breaths and then start to roll back up. This time, imagine each vertebra one at a time stacking back on top of the one below it, starting from your bottom vertebra and working up your back. Your head should be the last thing to come up and rest back on top of the stack.

Beginners – only roll part way down and begin seated before progressing to standing.

Advanced – once you are fully rolled down, experiment with moving your body to release it more – shift your weight from one foot to the other to deepen the stretch into the backs of your legs and turn your body gently from side to side.

General activity 3 (G3): Fascial squatting (good for everyone)

In Chapter 2 we talked a lot about the sitting epidemic that is contributing to many chronic pain conditions. Some people go so far as to call it "death by sitting." Whatever you think of sitting, if you think about it at all, it is not natural and it contributes to your body basically switching off as it no longer has to support itself.

The human body was never designed to sit at a 90 degree angle and prolonged sitting can lead to many postural changes, such as:

- Your buttocks switch off, which means they are no longer able to do their job in helping you to walk, run, jump, stand up, and sit down.
- Your abdominal muscles switch off too, which causes your posture to collapse in on itself.
- Your hips become less mobile, which means they are less able to do their job of stabilizing and balancing your body.
- Too much sitting and too little moving weakens your bones.
- Too much sitting also changes the posture in your hips and lower back, which puts more pressure on your discs and increases the risk of back pain and disc prolapse.

- Without getting too down and dirty, sitting on toilets is not natural either and actually pinches off the end of the colon so your bowels are unable to release properly.
- Sitting can also contribute to the development of many chronic conditions and diseases such as cardiac disease, high blood pressure, diabetes, and cancer.

So, if sitting is so bad for us, what is the answer? In many traditional cultures around the world, people squat instead of sit. They squat to rest, to cook, to work, and to defecate. In these cultures, back pain is almost non-existent, as are many of the digestive disorders common in the western world.

Squatting is a natural position which extends the lumbar spine and stretches the muscles and fascia in the lower back. The spine is not compressed and the weight of the body is evenly distributed between the legs, hips, and core. It also helps to increase the flexibility and health of the joints in the hips, knees, and ankles.

Squatting also helps to stretch and relax the pelvic floor. Contrary to popular belief, many people suffer from incontinence and conditions such as pelvic pain and prostatitis not because they have weak pelvic floor muscles, but actually because their pelvic floor is too tight and cannot contract and relax to support the pelvic organs.

By practicing squatting regularly you can help your body to undo many of the restrictions that have developed and will be contributing to your chronic pain condition, wherever you feel the pain. It is one of the most effective ways of returning your body to better balanced health and, like everything we suggest in this book, it is simple to do.

If you find the steps described below too difficult, then you can start by practicing horizontal squatting, that is lying on your back (Figure 11.15)! Lie on your back on the floor or your bed and bring your knees up to your chest. Just let them drop out to the sides

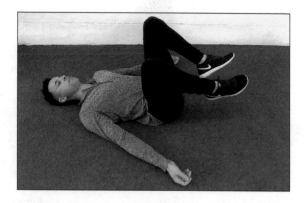

Figure 11.15: For complete beginners to squatting, this floor version is a great way of opening out the hips without also having to balance yourself.

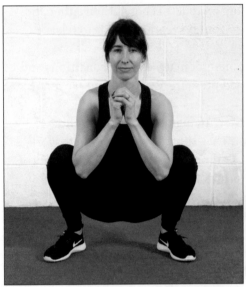

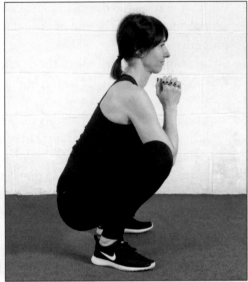

Figure 11.16: Fascial squat – keep your back straight and bottom dropped to allow the pelvic floor muscles to relax and help loosen the joints of the hips, knees and ankles.

Figure 11.17: Fascial squat seen from the side.

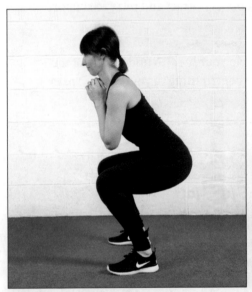

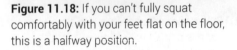

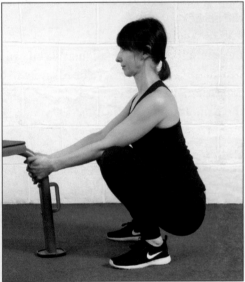

Figure 11.18: If you can't fully squat comfortably with your feet flat on the floor, this is a halfway position.

Figure 11.19: When you first start squatting, you might find you tip backwards as you drop your bottom down– to prevent this, hold onto a table leg or something similar.

and hang there. Doing this for at least 2 minutes will start to stretch the fascia in your hips and groin and you should feel a sensation of your legs releasing further. If this becomes uncomfortable, you can support your legs with pillows until your body gets used to the stretch. And then you can progress on to fascial squatting.

Top tips for sustained fascial squatting:

- Practice it daily. Start with just 1 minute (time it) and build up from there (Figure 11.16).
- Do not expect to be perfect when you start. Most people have such tight joints at first that they cannot get into a full squat. Instead, get down as far as is comfortable and progress from there (Figure 11.18).
- Keep your feet flat on the floor. Do not be tempted to raise your heels as this will not stretch anything properly.
- Keep your legs wide and point your toes out. The wider your stance, the further down you can get.
- Hold on to something. When you first start, you will have a tendency to fall over backwards until your body learns how to balance itself. Holding on to a table leg, door frame, or anything solid will help you to stay in a squat (Figure 11.19).
- Relax while you are down there. This might not be easy at first, but it will come as your body loosens more.
- If you have a problem with bowel movement, consider getting a footstool to use when you are sitting on the toilet. This helps by changing the angle of your lower back and pelvis, taking the pressure off your colon and making it easier to defecate without straining.

Beginners – practice horizontal squatting first.

Advanced – increase the time you squat and try using that time to do different things – adjusting your angles and rediscovering a sense of movement in your hips – make it a new healthy habit.

General activity 4 (G4): Fascial breathing (good for everyone)

First make sure that you are in a relaxed, quiet space and make yourself comfortable, whether seated or lying down. Tune in to your breath and notice where and how you are breathing. Are you breathing through your nose, your mouth, or both? Is your ribcage moving as you breathe, or does your breath feel tight and shallow?

When you first start to practice fascial breathing, it is a good idea to place the palms of your hands on your lower ribs (Figure 11.20). This way you can notice how your ribcage moves when you breathe. If your diaphragm is engaged, then your ribs will move out and slightly up towards your head as you breathe in, and then in and slightly down towards your feet as you breathe out. It is a good idea to practice this a few times before you start so you get the feeling in your hands and your body.

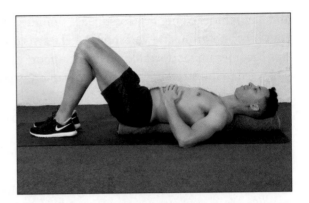

Figure 11.20: Fascial breathing is nice when combined with the towel stretch. Place your hands on your lower ribs to feel the rise and fall as you slowly breathe in and out.

Then start to breathe in a pattern of 7/11 breathing – breathe in for a count of 7 and then out for a count of 11, really emptying your lungs. When you finish breathing out, just allow yourself to be still for a moment before breathing in again. This still point encourages further deep relaxation in the body.

At first just practice fascial breathing for 5 minutes a day and gradually increase the time until you can manage 10 to 15 minutes. You can combine this with your towel stretch.

Beginners – if you find that you are struggling toward the end of either the in-breath or the out-breath, or if you feel you have to force the end of your out-breath, then simply shorten the count for both until you feel comfortable. The most important thing is that you feel comfortable and relaxed throughout, not forcing or rushing anything. And always keep the out-breath longer than the in-breath, as this helps to stimulate the rest and digest system.

Advanced – gradually increase the amount of time you practice fascial breathing each day.

General activity 5 (G5): Epsom salts baths (not good for pregnant women or people with sensitive skin)

Often the traditional ways are the best ways. Epsom salts is a very old remedy that helps to reduce aches and tensions in your body.

Epsom salts are bath salts that contain magnesium and sodium. The magnesium helps to relax the muscles, fascia, and other soft tissues in your body, and the sodium gently draws toxins and other waste products from your body.

Epsom salts are inexpensive and can be purchased from most independent chemists or online. Add two handfuls to a hot bath and soak in the bath for 20 minutes – this is also a good excuse for some "me time."

If you do not have a bath tub, try an Epsom salts foot bath – just put a handful of the salts into a bowl of hot water and soak your feet for 20 minutes. This will also help to relax the rest of your body.

Having an Epsom salts bath or foot bath before bed can help to relax your mind–body and help with a good night's sleep.

Fascial stretches and how to do them

Fascial stretches are designed to stretch the body along fascial lines of tension. If you need motivation, it is worth reading and re-reading the section "How to stretch" as it explains the links between fascial anatomy, chronic pain, and the benefits of fascial stretching.

Why stretch?

Stretching is so important, so natural, and such a lovely thing to do, but so many of us regard it as something to rush through at the beginning or end of an exercise routine. Many people skip stretching altogether and, of the people left, most are not doing it in a way that will give them lasting benefit. But stretching is an easy exercise activity in itself and can bring significant health benefits. For anyone with limited movement through injury and chronic pain, stretching is a brilliant way to start reclaiming your pain-free fascial health.

There are also so many different types of stretching that people can get confused about what stretches are best for them. Terms like "isometric," "assisted," "resistance," "active isolated," and "ballistic" stretches are bandied around in the sports fitness world. Each is effective in a particular situation, but these stretches are focused on muscles when what is needed is a fascial perspective.

The muscular approach means stretching an individual muscle or group of muscles for 20 to 30 seconds per stretch. This is enough time for the muscle fibers to stretch and let go of some of their tension. If practiced regularly and mindfully, muscle stretches can help to loosen tight muscles and restricted joints, and they can improve posture, flexibility and circulation as well as decreasing the risk of injury and muscle soreness after exercise.

However, as we have seen already (Chapter 5), muscles are not the be-all and end-all movement makers we may once have thought. Most movement occurs via functional units of fascia that coordinate direction and energy release; and most body–mind tension is held in the fascia.

When not to stretch

Almost everyone can stretch fascially and safely from day one. However, there are two categories of people who may need to work up to it or do something else to help their fascia. These are:

*   anyone who is jammed into whole-body systemic pain at the moment
*   anyone who is hypermobile (you will know if you are).

Sometimes people with chronic pain find it difficult to stretch at all. This can be because the fascia throughout their body is so stuck, so restricted, and so sensitive that even the slightest stretch can trigger a disproportionately large systemic pain response. (This is not to be confused with a general reluctance to try, a little wariness and caution, or limited local pain, all of which affect most of us from time to time.)

If you find that this applies to you, then maybe your body is not ready to stretch just yet. There are other techniques you can use to help calm your pain response and remind your body that it can move, such as the general activities described above. It is perfectly realistic to stay optimistic. Remember, the natural state of the body is fluid, pain-free movement and this can be achieved with a little patience and your new fascial understanding.

Some people are hypermobile, which means that their joints can move beyond a normal range of movement. Hypermobile people tend to be very bendy, they can stretch easily, and they can often do "party tricks" such as bending their thumbs back to touch their wrists. They can do this is because their collagen is different, so tissues that would normally be strong, such as the joint capsules, ligaments, and tendons that support joints, are more elastic and their joints can be easily displaced or dislocated.

To compensate for the laxity in these structures, and to keep the body stable, the muscles and fascia surrounding the affected joints tighten more than usual and can get stuck. This constant tightening causes the muscles to become tired and weak which then causes pain and stiffness. Many hypermobile people also have a weaker than normal sense of proprioception (see Chapter 5) and therefore tend to bump into things or drop things. As a result, they also have a greater tendency to injure themselves.

Stretching, even fascial stretching, is of no benefit to hypermobile people as they can usually stretch themselves to beyond a normal range of movement even when their tissues are tight. In fact, stretching can actually do them more harm than good.

A hypermobile person will get more benefit from releasing the muscles and fascia between the joints (rather than around them), using the myofascial ball work exercises (see below) and practicing a movement therapy such as Pilates or Alexander technique that will strengthen their core and improve their posture. This will balance the pressure on specific joints, improve proprioception and coordination, strengthen and tone muscles, and take the pressure off the fascia, allowing it to naturally return to a position of better equilibrium.

With those two exceptions in mind, everyone else can get on and enjoy self-help through fascial stretching.

How to stretch your fascia

We learned about fascial anatomy in Chapter 5. Here is where our new-found knowledge comes alive.

Just as muscles are arranged in local fascial units designed to coordinate movement, so the whole body works along fascial lines of tension, intended to maintain balance. Knowing this gives us a totally new way to think about stretching. Instead of thinking about stretching individual muscles, we can stretch our fascia along these known lines of fascial tension. Doing this enables the fascia to release and the effects to be communicated throughout the body.

The representation of the fascial lines of tension in Figures 11.21–24 were developed by Tom Myers. They show how injury in one area can affect a totally different part of the body, but more importantly here, how a single stretch can benefit the whole body.

Much like fascial anatomy requires you to unlearn some of what you thought you knew, so fascial stretching asks you to throw away the stretching book and discard everything you have ever been taught about muscle stretches. Fascial stretching is a whole new way of stretching and letting go, one that is gentler on your body and more deeply effective.

The first thing to unlearn is that you do not need to repeat lots of short stretches. A typical muscle fiber will release in 20 to 30 seconds, which is why muscle stretches are short. However, fascia responds to slower, gentler pressure (remember thixotrophy from Chapter 5). Fascia takes around 90 to 120 seconds (1½ minutes to 2 minutes) to start to release. Holding one single stretch for 2 to 5 minutes will allow additional fascial releases to occur throughout the body. Remembering that everything is connected to everything else; the longer you hold a stretch, the further it will release in a three-dimensional response transmitted through the fascial web.

When you start fascial stretching it may take a little time to get a sense of how long 2 to 5 minutes really is. This is because we are often focused on conscious counting rather that going with the fascial feel of the stretch. The easiest way to solve this is to use a timer – set it for 2 minutes at first to give your mind–body the chance to learn what 2 minutes feels like. You are then free to follow and enjoy the sensations of fascial stretches as they work through your fascia. Eventually you will be able to stretch for 2 to 5 minutes without the need for a timer.

Next, you can unlearn the rule that says you need to stretch both sides. You were almost certainly taught to do a set of 10 short muscle stretches on one side immediately followed by a set of 10 on the opposite side. This will not stretch your fascia and it is unnecessary in fascial stretching. First, fast repetitions will not do anything to stretch your fascia; you will just be demonstrating your muscle's tendency to bounce straight back into problem postures unless you take the time to stretch your fascia. Second, in the fascial world, one stretch can connect throughout your body, making it unnecessary to stretch both sides unless, of course, you would like to.

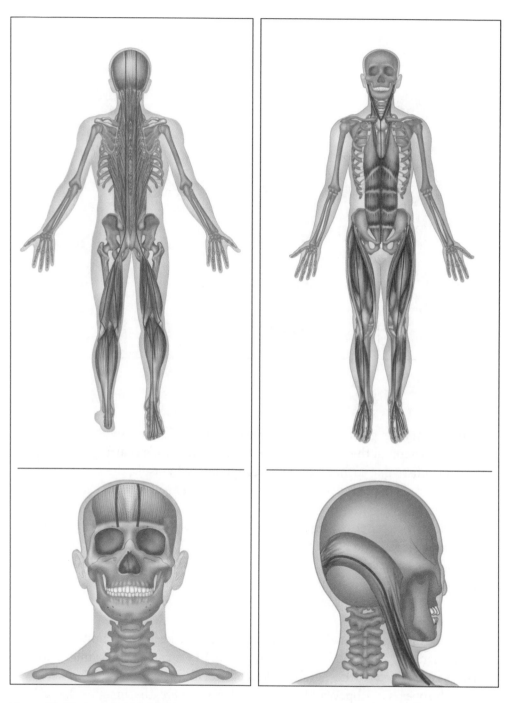

Figure 11.21: Superficial back line.

Figure 11.22: Superficial front line.

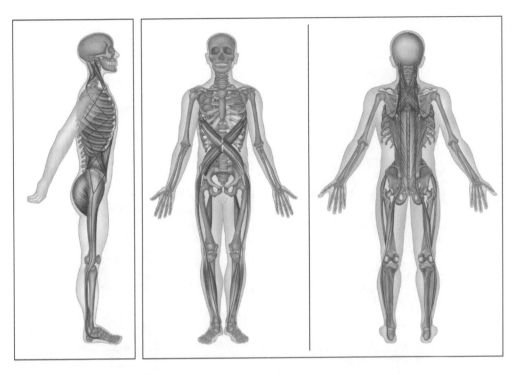

Figure 11.23: Lateral (side) line.

Figure 11.24: Spiral line – front and back.

The third point to let go of is that stretching is an optional extra, something to be done half-heartedly at the beginning or end of a routine while chatting to your mates at the gym or listening to music on your headphones. Physically, there is nothing to stop you stretching fascia in this way, but you will not get as much benefit as you will by actually paying attention to your fascia while you stretch. From an energetic point of view (Chapter 5), paying attention to any body tissue or part of your body will encourage it respond better to what you want it to do. Mindful fascial stretching will encourage more stretching and release in the tissue. However, this does not mean that you have to stretch in monastic silence. You can always play some relaxing music in the background if you find this helps.

As you move into a stretch, take it slowly, do not try to take it to the limit straight away. Instead, pay attention to what is happening in your stretch. You might notice yourself pause as you reach what feels like a barrier (a fascial restriction), where the stretch appears to stop. Wait here, remembering to breathe, imagine the gentle internal pressure of the stretch elongating the tissues and melting the fascia until it releases and the stretch can move on. Allow your stretch to continue slowly until you meet the next restriction and, again, pause here breathing deeply, feeling the gentle pressure allowing it to release.

You may notice different sensations as each restriction releases. Sometimes you might feel localized tension and pulling, or a softening and lengthening in your tissues. Other possible sensations can be a ripping sensation like Velcro separating, or warmth, tingling, pulsing, and gentle twitching. Sensations of localized pain can intensify and then fall away. These are all the feelings of fascial restrictions letting go, releasing.

The more mindful you are of what your body is doing, the more it will release. This takes practice, but you will start to feel more sensations as you work. Often as one release happens, you will feel a niggle or sensation in another part of your body which tells you where to stretch next.

Sometimes people say they cannot feel anything happening. If you are stretching your fascia for at least 90 to 120 seconds, then something will definitely be happening and you will soon feel the benefit, although you may have to wait a while until you tune in and start to feel the process.

Going back to mindful stretching, if it helps to soothe you in these early stages, you can always choose a little relaxing background music to keep you company during your self-help stretching session, just choose something appropriate – blasting out high energy tunes will do nothing to help your fascia relax.

Just as myofascial release therapy can trigger unwinding, so can fascial stretching. A general principle in myofascial release therapy is that it is always good to follow, but not force, an unwinding release. This applies equally to self-help fascial stretching. Sometimes during a stretch you might feel like you just want to add an extra degree of twist or another inch of stretch to follow the release. When this happens go with the flow, "listen" with your whole mind–body, and follow your fascia. Not only will this feel a whole lot better, it can be exciting and enjoyable to follow your fascia on its journey of unwinding, as stretch becomes movement.

As you get to the end of each fascial stretch, remember to come out of it gently and gradually, and then spend a few seconds relaxing. Maybe jiggle around with all the other atoms – shake out your limbs or just do your thang. Moving like this will help to reinforce the releases that have just occurred, let go of energy, and prepare your body for the next stretch.

Finally, an additional benefit of fascial stretching is that, as well as letting go of restrictions, you are also strengthening your muscles at the same time, helping to settle imbalances into healthy new postures. As you stretch out along fascial lines the muscles that support that stretch must contract, giving them new tone, and strength.

Fascial stretch 1 (S1): Neck and arms

Standing or sitting, slowly take your head to the side, bringing your ear towards your shoulder. Allow your arms to hang by your sides and keep your arms and shoulders loose (Figure 11.25).

As with all fascial stretches, gently move deeper into the stretch, waiting when you feel barriers and slowly breathing into them to allow deeper release. Imagine your opposite arm elongating and stretching away from your neck to create a three-dimensional fascial stretch in a pattern from your fingers to your arm, neck, and head.

Beginners – it is a good idea to practice this by looking into a mirror at first, as many people have a tendency to raise their shoulders up as they stretch (Figure 11.26).

Advanced – to deepen the stretch place your hand on the side of your head, but do not force it; only use the pressure of your hand as a counterweight (Figure 11.27).

Fascial stretch 2 (S2): Neck and back

Standing or sitting, drop your head forwards onto your chest and turn it so that your nose is pointing towards your armpit. As this stretch develops you will feel the releases moving down your neck into your shoulder and down your back (Figures 11.28 and 11.29).

Beginners – as you drop your head forward, allow it to roll gently from side to side across your chest to help loosen the tissues in your neck before going into the stretch.

Advanced – as you go into the stretch, and if it is comfortable for you, bring your hand up onto the top of your head and apply gentle downward pressure to increase the stretch. Again, do not use your hand to force the stretch (Figure 11.30).

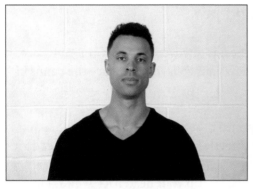

Figure 11.25: The start position for the neck and arm stretch S1 with your head level.

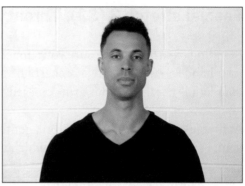

Figure 11.28: The start position for the neck and back stretch S2 with your head level.

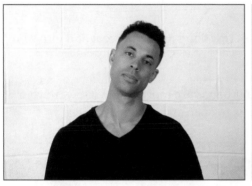

Figure 11.26: Tilt your head to take your ear towards your shoulder until you feel a stretch in your neck. Practice this in a mirror at first to check your shoulders don't lift as you stretch.

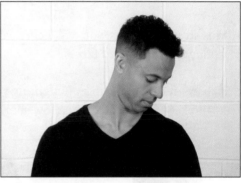

Figure 11.29: Turn your head to one side and drop it down so your nose is pointing at your armpit. You will feel a stretch in the back of the opposite shoulder.

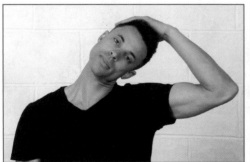

Figure 11.27: If it feels comfortable, you can use your hand to deepen the stretch, being mindful not to overstretch your fascia.

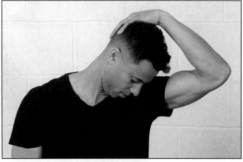

Figure 11.30: If it feels comfortable, you can use your hand to deepen the stretch, being mindful not to overstretch your fascia.

Fascial stretch 3 (S3): Throat and jaw

Standing or sitting, make sure your upper chest is uncovered so that you can place your hands on the skin of your chest just below your collarbones. Place the palms of your hands here, with your arms crossed.

At first just allow your hands to sink gently onto the skin; imagine they are making contact with the superficial fascia which is directly below the skin and attached to it.

Once you can feel (or imagine) that contact, slowly tip your head back while gently pulling your hands downwards. Your hands should stay where they are and not slide on your skin, and you should feel a sensation of stretching of the skin on your throat. It is best to relax your jaw and open your mouth, to prevent any tension in your jaw.

As this stretch deepens, you will feel releases travelling up your throat and into your jaw, mouth, tongue, and face.

Beginners – feel the stretch by imagining your hands are moving down toward your feet, and keep your head level. Allow your jaw to open and soften (Figure 11.31).

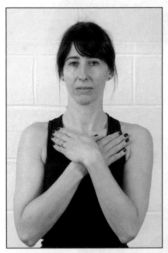 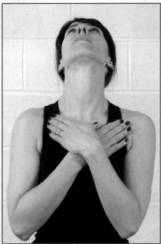 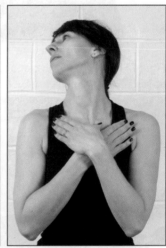

Figure 11.31: Cross your hands on your chest just under your collarbones. Your hands should be directly on skin. Gently pull your hands down while keeping your jaw relaxed.

Figure 11.32: For a deeper stretch, tip your head back and pull your hands gently down until you feel a stretch in your throat.

Figure 11.33: Turn your head gradually to the side to feel a stretch into the side of your neck and ear.

Advanced – experiment by gently and slowly turning your head from side to side to feel the releases extending into the sides of your jaw and your ears (Figure 11.33).

Fascial stretch 4 (S4): Arms and hands

You can either do these stretches sitting or kneeling, whichever is most comfortable for you.

If sitting, position yourself in front of a desk or table and make sure you can comfortably touch the edge with your wrists, keeping your arms straight. Keep your feet on the floor to steady yourself.

For the first position, straighten your arms and place your fingers on the edge of the desk/table, so that your palms are facing the edge (Figures 11.34 and 11.35). Stretch your arms towards the desk/table until you feel a stretch in the underside of your forearms. Adjust the pressure so that you can remain in a comfortable stretch and allow this stretch to deepen as the tissues start to relax and release. Keep your shoulders and neck relaxed and loose.

For the second position, turn your hands over and place the backs of your hands against the desk/table (Figures 11.36 and 11.37). Stretch your arms towards the desk/table until you feel a stretch in the tops of your forearms. Adjust the pressure as above.

If kneeling on the floor, place your hands palm down on the floor. Gently lean forward until you feel a stretch in the underside of your forearms (Figures 11.38 and 11.39).

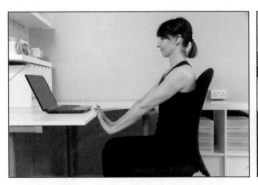

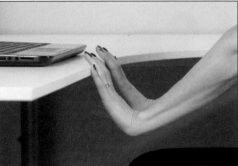

Figure 11.34: S4 – seated at a desk, rest your fingers against the desk edge, keeping your shoulders relaxed.

Figure 11.35: Close-up of hands – the aim is to feel a stretch into the underside of your forearms.

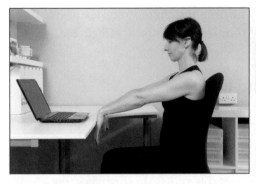

Figure 11.36: Seated at a desk, rest the backs of your hands against the desk edge, keeping your shoulders relaxed.

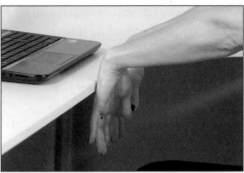

Figure 11.37: Close-up of hands – the aim is to feel a stretch into the tops of your forearms.

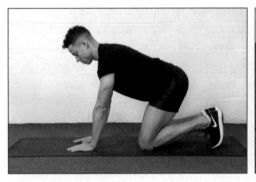

Figure 11.38: S4 – kneeling, place the palms of your hands on the floor, keeping your shoulders relaxed.

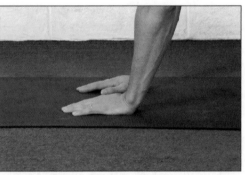

Figure 11.39: Close-up of hands – the aim is to feel a stretch into the underside of your forearms.

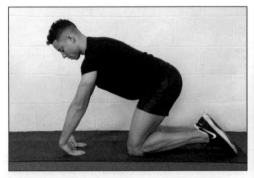

Figure 11.40: Kneeling, place the backs of your hands on the floor, keeping your shoulders relaxed.

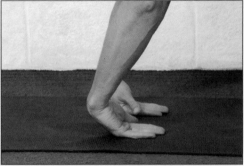

Figure 11.41: Close-up of hands – the aim is to feel a stretch into the tops of your forearms.

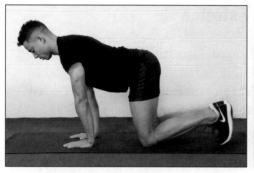

Figure 11.42: From this position, lean your weight forward slightly to deepen the stretch into the underside of your forearms.

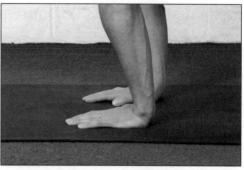

Figure 11.43: Close-up of hands – adjust your weight to increase the stretch.

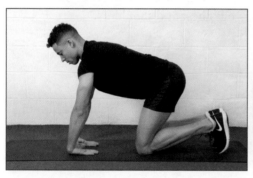

Figure 11.44: From this position, lean your weight back slightly to deepen the stretch into the tops of your forearms.

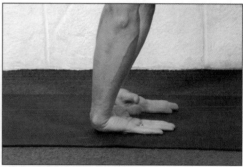

Figure 11.45: Close-up of hands – adjust your weight to increase the stretch.

Adjust the pressure so that you can remain in a comfortable stretch and allow this stretch to deepen as the tissues start to relax and release. Keep your shoulders and neck relaxed and loose.

For the second position, turn your hands over and place your arms in front of you with the backs of your hands on the floor (Figures 11.40 and 11.41). Gently lean back until you feel a stretch in the tops of your forearms. Adjust the pressure as above.

Beginners – just the pressure of the stretches will be enough without leaning into these stretches. If the kneeling version is too intense, try the stretches against a wall instead.

Advanced – as you lean into the stretches, experiment with changing angle and moving your body to feel releases in different areas of your arms and hands (Figures 11.42–11.45).

Fascial stretch 5 (S5): Doorway stretch

Find a convenient doorway that is not being used. Place your hands on either side of the door frame so your palms are resting on it with your arms bent. Take a step through the doorway to feel a stretch across the front of your chest. Do not force the stretch, just allow your body to lean forward as the fascia releases and the stretch deepens (Figure 11.46).

Beginners – stand to one side of a doorway, place your shoulder and arm against the door frame and twist your body away from the door frame. You should feel the stretch in your chest (Figures 11.47 and 11.48).

Advanced – try moving your hands to different positions higher and lower on the door frame to stretch into different areas in your chest and shoulders.

Fascial stretch 6 (S6): Sides

Sitting or standing, slowly lean your body over to one side, with a feeling of hinging at your waist. As you lean, take a deep breath in and, as you exhale, feel the side of your ribcage expanding and lengthening (Figures 11.49 and 11.50).

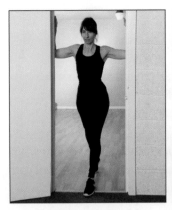

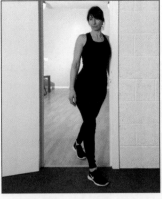

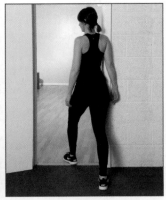

Figure 11.46: S5 – place hands on either side of the doorframe and take a step through to feel a stretch across your chest.

Figure 11.47: For a stretch without using your arms, place your shoulder against the doorframe and twist your body away.

Figure 11.48: Beginners' doorway stretch seen from the back.

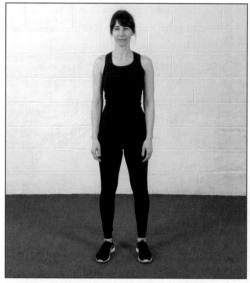

Figure 11.49: Start position for side stretch S6 with your body level.

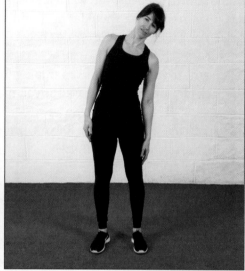

Figure 11.50: Lean your upper body to the side, keeping your arms loose, to feel a stretch into your side.

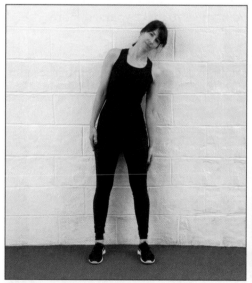

Figure 11.51: You can do this stretch against a wall – maintain contact between your back and the wall to stop your upper body from twisting forward.

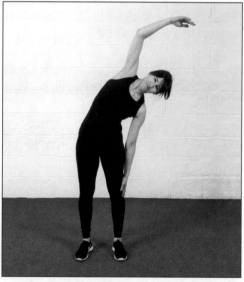

Figure 11.52: To deepen the stretch, take your arm over your head.

As the stretch deepens, you will feel releases extending down into your hip and leg, and up into your ribs, shoulder neck and arm. Imagine the two-way stretch creating space along the whole side of your body.

Beginners – to stop yourself from tipping forwards, keep your back leaning against the back of your chair or the wall as you move into the stretch (Figure 11.51).

Advanced – if it is comfortable for you, bring your arm up and over your head to deepen the stretch (Figure 11.52).

Fascial stretch 7 (S7): Spinal twist

Lie on your back on the floor or on your bed with your knees bent (Figure 11.53). Gently allow your knees to drop over to one side. As you do, stretch your arms out to the sides and ensure that you keep both shoulder blades in contact with the floor/bed (Figure 11.54). To deepen the stretch, turn your head in the opposite direction from your legs.

Beginners – if you find your legs do not make contact with the floor/bed and are dangling in space, put a pillow underneath your knees to make yourself more comfortable (Figure 11.55).

Advanced – try extending your top leg out straight to deepen the stretch into the sides of your hips and buttocks (Figure 11.56).

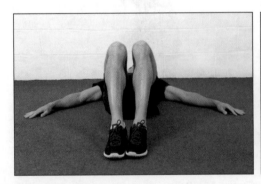

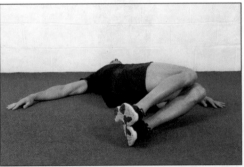

Figure 11.53: Start position for the spinal twist S7, lie on the floor with your knees bent and head level.

Figure 11.54: Take your legs to one side, keeping your head level, and both shoulders in contact with the floor.

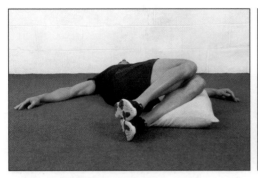

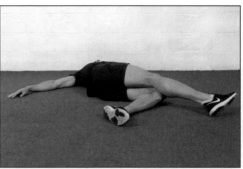

Figure 11.55: If the full stretch is uncomfortable, place a pillow under your knees to support your legs.

Figure 11.56: To deepen the stretch, straighten your top leg, and turn your head in the opposite direction to your legs.

Fascial stretch 8 (S8): Front of hips

Move into a kneeling lunge position, with one knee on the floor and the other leg straight out behind you. You might want to put a small pillow under your knee (Figure 11.57). Make sure you keep your upper body upright by resting your hands on your thigh and do not slump forward as you stretch.

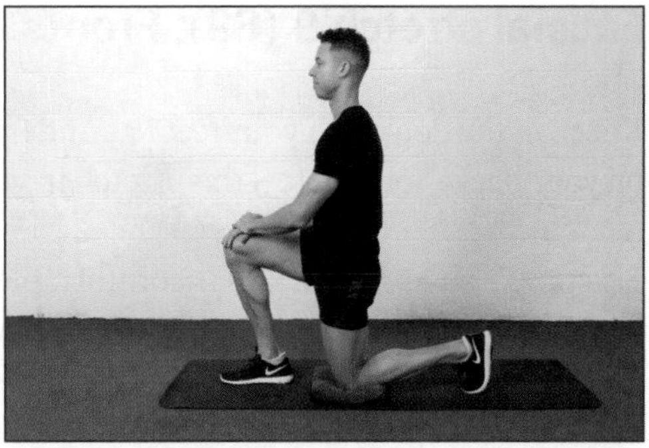

Beginners – if kneeling is not a comfortable position, try lying on a bed or a sturdy table and allow one leg to drop off the side – your foot can either make contact with the floor or, for a deeper stretch, lie on something high enough to allow your leg to hang freely (Figure 11.58).

Figure 11.57: S8 – kneel on one knee, keeping your upper body straight and support your hands on your leg. Place a small cushion under your knee for comfort.

Advanced – to deepen this stretch you can lean your weight forwards, while keeping your upper body upright (Figure 11.59).

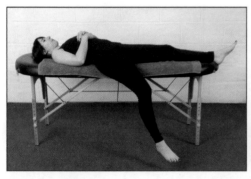

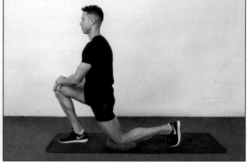

Figure 11.58: Lie on your bed or a sturdy table and drop one leg off – your foot can be touching the floor if this is more comfortable.

Figure 11.59: To deepen the stretch, lean your weight forward while keeping your upper body upright.

Fascial stretch 9 (S9): Fronts of legs and feet

Kneel on the floor with your feet flat underneath you and lean back to rest your bottom on your heels. You will feel this stretch in your thighs, shins and feet (Figure 11.60).

Beginners – sit as far back as is comfortable on your heels – if necessary place a pillow between your calves and bottom (Figure 11.61).

Advanced – deepen the stretch by leaning your upper body further back and support yourself with your arms (Figure 11.62).

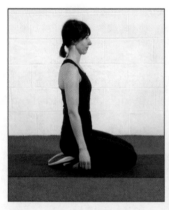

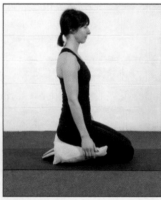

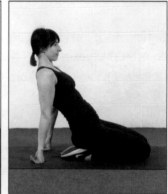

Figure 11.60: Kneel on the floor with both feet flat under you. Keep your upper body upright.

Figure 11.61: If your knees feel uncomfortable in the full stretch, place a pillow between your bottom and legs for support.

Figure 11.62: To deepen the stretch, lean back and support yourself with your arms.

Fascial stretch 10 (S10): Back of legs and feet

Find a convenient step or use an exercise step. Face into the step with your heels positioned backwards off the edge. Allow both heels to drop down to feel a stretch into the back of both legs from the soles of your feet, up through your ankles, calves and into your hamstrings and back. Support yourself with your hand against a wall if necessary (Figures 11.63 and 11.64).

Beginners – keep both feet level to feel a stretch in the back of your legs (Figures 11.65 and 11.66).

Advanced – drop one heel down to feel a deeper stretch into the back of your leg (Figures 11.67 and 11.68).

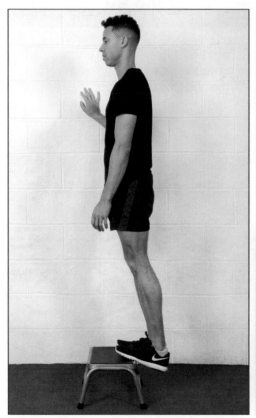

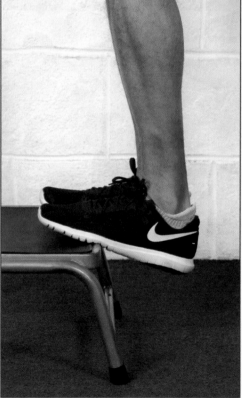

Figure 11.63: S10 – standing on a step, drop both heels down.

Figure 11.64: Close-up of foot position – the aim is to feel an equal stretch in both legs.

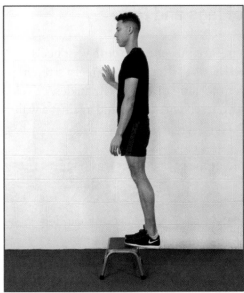

Figure 11.65: Standing on a step with both heels extended out, keeping your feet level.

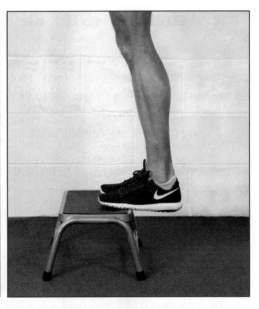

Figure 11.66: Close-up of foot position – you can keep your balance by adjusting how far your heels extend off the step.

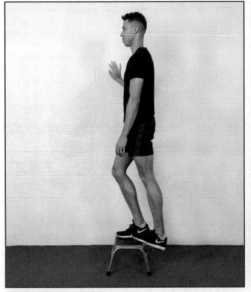

Figure 11.67: For a deeper stretch, drop one heel down.

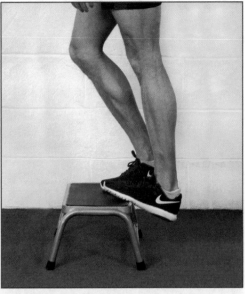

Figure 11.68: Close-up of foot position – the aim is to feel a deeper stretch in your calf and hamstrings.

Myofascial ball work and how to do the myofascial ball exercises

These myofascial ball work exercises are great for working on specific areas of myofascial tension and trigger points in muscles. They require use of one or two suitable balls. I recommend a myofascial ball kit, which has specifically been designed for this purpose. Please read the section below on using myofascial balls before starting the exercises.

Using myofascial balls

People sometimes use one or two balls as an accessory to help with self-myofascial release, and this can be extremely beneficial.

The benefit of using balls is that they can help you apply the necessary gentle pressure to hard-to-reach places. And some conditions lend themselves really well to this. For example, a runner with plantar fasciitis affecting the arch of the foot can work on this area while seated by rolling the ball around under their foot and up the lower leg in the directions that feel good and help to release the restrictions.

Many people improvise using different types of ball – I have heard of anything from a spiky massage ball to a cricket ball! While these can provide some relief, it can be difficult to relax your weight and still achieve the gentle yielding pressure that is necessary for fascial release. I recommend a myofascial release ball kit that is made for the purpose.

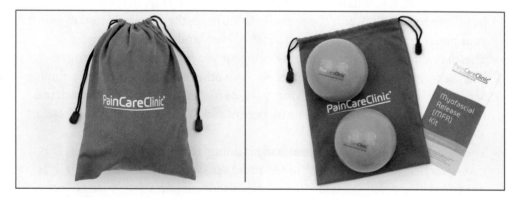

Figure 11.69: The Myofascial Release (MFR) Kit.

The ideal is an inflatable PVC ball around 10 cm in diameter, which is large enough to cover a good area yet still small enough to focus in on irritable spots. An inflatable ball is softer and therefore more giving than other balls and can be inflated or deflated to suit the sensitivity of your tissues. When your restrictions are tight or your body is hypersensitive, as, for example, with fibromyalgia, a softer pressure is required at first to encourage your fascia to let go.

You can use myofascial balls on any area of your body and may need one or two balls depending on where you are working. When you use two balls it is best to have a pouch to keep them stable, otherwise you may find that one pops out from under you when you apply any pressure! You can purchase a specially designed myofascial ball kit that includes two balls and a pouch, enabling you to use the balls safely and easily in any area of your body.

The principles of using myofascial release balls are the same as everything else fascial:

- Before you start to use the ball(s), tune in to your fascial body first and check where you are feeling restrictions, tension, or pain. This will be a good place to start.
- You can either lie on a ball, wedge it against a wall and lean against it, or sit and use it elsewhere on your body, depending on where you want to work.
- If you are comfortable working on the floor, then this is best because it is a hard surface that resists and reflects the pressure of a ball well. However, if you find this is too much, or you have difficulty getting down to or up from the floor, then you can lie on your bed to use the ball(s).
- Once in position, relax your body around the ball(s) (supporting yourself with pillows or cushions if necessary). The idea is to feel a gentle but consistent pressure that you can relax into so your tissues can start to soften and melt as they release. If you have to hold tension in your body just to maintain your position on the ball(s), or if the pressure is too hard, then you will need to adjust your position until you can achieve a stable, even, and gentle pressure.
- This may simply feel like the pain reducing, or you might feel a softening or lengthening of the tissues in the area, or even other sensations such as a ripping sensation, warmth, tingling, pulsing, pain, or melting. Sometimes you will feel the sensations intensify as the release occurs and then they fade away. These are all signals of fascial release.
- The more you tune in to what your body is doing, the more it will release. This takes practice, but you will start to feel more sensations as you work. Often, as one release happens, you will feel a niggle or sensation in another part of your body; this tells you where to work next.

- Because this is fascial work and everything is connected to everything else, it is not necessary to work on both sides of your body. So you do not need to work on your left hip just because you have worked on your right hip. Your body will automatically shift, rebalance and settle as the fascial release happens.
- As with fascial stretching, you may not feel anything much happening, but rest assured that if you are holding gentle pressure in one place for at least 90 to 120 seconds this will be triggering a release in the tissues. Sometimes some areas are so restricted that it takes a few sessions for them to start to let go, and for you to start to feel that response.
- It is quite usual for work of this sort to be accompanied by internal sensation, involuntary movement, or perhaps reddening of the skin. These are all signs of fascial release and are to be welcomed.
- Little and regular is far more helpful that a lengthy and intense session, particularly as you get used to working with myofascial balls.

Myofascial ball work 1 (B1): Back of neck

The back of the neck is a fantastic area to release for many chronic pain conditions. It helps with neck and shoulder pain, headaches and migraines, and RSI symptoms in the arms and hands. Because using the balls in this area releases fascial restrictions in the back of the neck, it can also help with back pain and some people can feel releases in their hips and legs. Releases here also help to release pressure on the vagus nerve, improving breathing, heart function, and digestion.

Position the MFR Kit just below the base of the skull with the balls on either side of your spine and rest the top of your head on a small pillow for support. Then allow your weight to sink onto the balls (Figure 11.70).

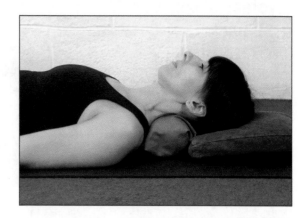

Figure 11.70: B1 – lie on your back on the floor with the MFR Kit under your neck. The balls should be positioned on either side of your spine. Support the top of your head with a small cushion for comfort.

Myofascial ball work 2 (B2): Side of neck

The side of the neck is an area where the nerves for the arms exit from the spinal cord and it can often become tight and restricted, especially in people who use computers a lot. Releasing this area can help with arm and hand pain, as well as more general neck, shoulder, and headache pains.

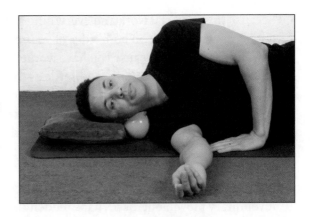

Figure 11.71: B2 – lie on your side with an MFR ball positioned on the side of your neck. Support your head with a small cushion for comfort.

Lie on your side and place one ball on the floor or bed, resting the side of your neck on it. You may need to place a small pillow under your head for support and comfort. Be careful not to place the ball too far forwards otherwise it will start to put pressure on your throat. Allow your bodyweight to sink into the ball, allowing an even pressure on the side of the neck (Figure 11.71).

Myofascial ball work 3 (B3): Back

Using the balls on your back can help with many pain conditions including back, neck, shoulder, and hip pains.

You can use the MFR Kit anywhere on your back, from the base of your neck all the way down to your lower back (Figures 11.72–11.74). And you can lie on the floor or a bed, depending on which is

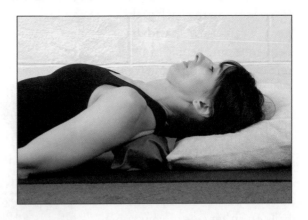

Figure 11.72: B3 – place the MFR Kit under your upper back between your shoulder blades. Position the balls either side of your spine. Support your head with a pillow for comfort.

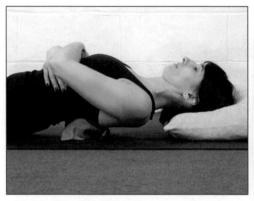

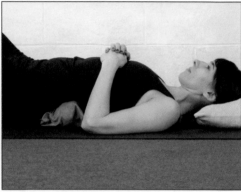

Figure 11.73: Place the MFR Kit under your mid-back. Position the balls either side of your spine. Support your head with a pillow for comfort. Allow your arms to relax by your sides (model has arms raised only to show Kit position in this picture).

Figure 11.74: Place the MFR Kit under your lower back. Position the balls either side of your spine. Support your head with a pillow for comfort and keep your legs bent. Allow your arms to relax by your side (model has arms raised only to show Kit position in this picture).

more comfortable for you. When you use the Kit on your back, just make sure your spine is positioned in the dip between the balls – pressure directly on your spine can be uncomfortable and prevent your body from relaxing.

Myofascial ball work 4 (B4): Armpits

Using a ball in your armpit is a fantastic way to release restrictions causing arm and hand pain, shoulder issues, and neck pain.

Lie on your side on the floor or bed, stretch your arm over your head and place the ball on the back of your armpit. Depending on where you position the ball, you will feel different sensations and you can gradually work your way from the top to the bottom of the area (Figure 11.75).

It often helps to place a pillow under your head to make yourself more comfortable.

If you have restricted shoulder movement, for example frozen shoulder symptoms, you can still place the ball along the side of your armpit without stretching your arm over your head (Figure 11.76).

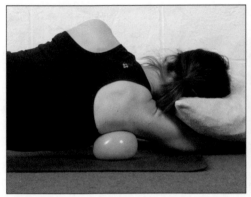

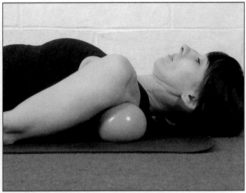

Figure 11.75: B4 – lying on your side, place the ball under your armpit with your arm positioned above your shoulder – you should feel the ball is on the outside edge of your shoulder blade. Support your head with a pillow for comfort.

Figure 11.76: This modified position can be used if you have any shoulder restrictions that make it uncomfortable to lie on your side or have your arm raised above your shoulder. Lie on your back with the ball under the back of your shoulder. Support your head with a small cushion for comfort if necessary.

Myofascial ball work 5 (B5): Arms

To work on your forearms, place the ball on a hard surface such as a table top. While standing, roll your forearm slowly and mindfully over the surface of the ball, stopping to allow releases where things feel tight or tender.

First, work on one side of the forearm from your elbow down to your wrist and then turn over your arm to work on the other side, moving your forearm over the ball (Figures 11.77–11.80).

Myofascial ball work 6 (B6): Hands

Our hands are active every day as we type, hold things, twist, and apply pressure using them. This causes the fascia in the palms of the hands to tighten and can contribute to RSI pains and conditions such as trigger finger. Being full of proprioceptors, our palms and fingers are also very sensitive so fascial restrictions in our hands can also contribute to clumsiness so we find it difficult to properly grasp and hold onto things without dropping them.

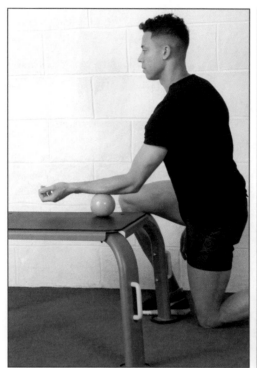 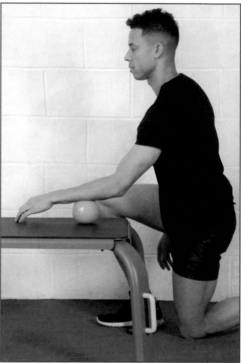

Figure 11.77: B5 – place the ball on a desk, table or kitchen counter and rest the back of your forearm on it. Make sure you are comfortable standing, sitting or kneeling, your hand, forearm and shoulders should be relaxed.

Figure 11.79: Place the ball on a desk, table or kitchen counter and rest the front of your forearm on it. Make sure you are comfortable standing, sitting or kneeling, your hand, forearm and shoulders should be relaxed.

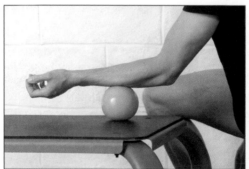 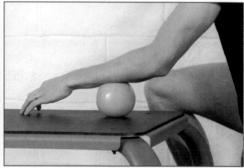

Figure 11.78: Close-up – you can slowly roll the ball under your forearm to work on different areas.

Figure 11.80: Close-up – you can slowly roll the ball under your forearm to work on different areas.

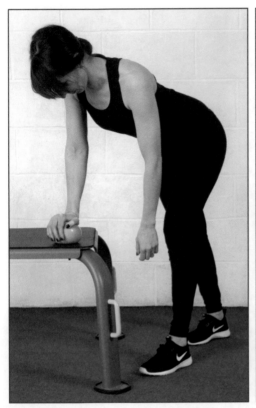

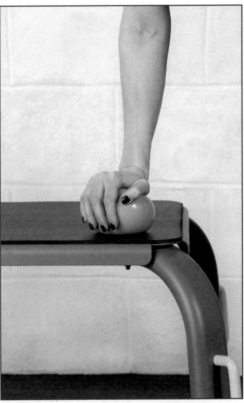

Figure 11.81: B6 – place the ball on a table, desk or kitchen counter and rest your hand on top. You should be able to comfortably lean into the ball without any stress on your upper body. Allow your other arm to hang loosely and keep your shoulders relaxed.

Figure 11.82: Close-up – you can slowly roll your hand over the ball to work on different areas.

To work on your hands, place the ball on a hard surface such as a table top. While standing, roll the palm of your hand over the surface of the ball very slowly and mindfully. Pay attention to where things feel tender or restricted and pause on these areas allowing a gentle pressure to accumulate until they release. You can roll onto your fingers and wrist too, allowing time for these areas to also let go (Figures 11.81 and 11.82).

As you work, be mindful to maintain your balance. Do not hold onto anything or rest your other hand on the table, but just keep it hanging loosely by your side, and allow your body to move and rebalance as the fascia in your hand releases.

Not only will the fascia on your hand loosen, the fascia all the way up your arm into your shoulder and neck will also start to loosen.

Myofascial ball work 7 (B7): Buttocks

To use the ball on your buttocks, you can sit, lie, or lean against a wall (Figures 11.83–11.87). The buttocks can be quite tight and painful, especially in anyone who has back, hip, or leg issues. This is because the sciatic nerve passes through here on its way from the spine to the leg. Therefore, care should be taken when using the ball in this area. If you feel an intense electric pain and your leg starts to feel a bit numb, then you are directly on the sciatic nerve and should move off to avoid irritating it.

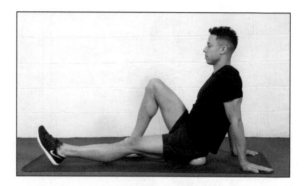

Figure 11.83: B7 – sitting on the floor, or on a seat, place the ball under your buttock. If on the floor, make sure your body is comfortably supported.

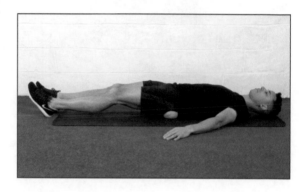

Figure 11.84: Alternatively you can lie on the floor with the ball placed under your buttock. Keep your body relaxed.

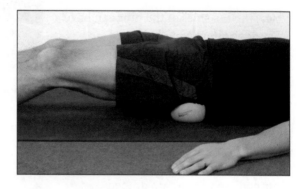

Figure 11.85: Close-up – allow your body time to soften onto the ball.

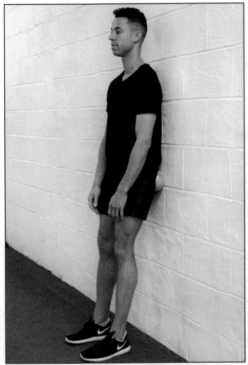

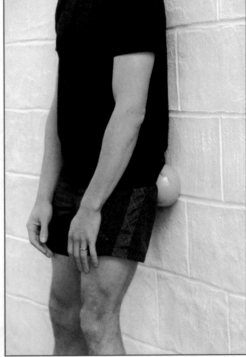

Figure 11.86: Alternatively you can lean yourself and the ball against a wall. Again make sure your body is relaxed and comfortable.

Figure 11.87: Close-up – allow your body time to soften onto the ball.

Myofascial ball work 8 (B8): Side of hips

Releasing the sides of the hips can have a beneficial impact on back and leg mobility, reducing pain in the back, buttocks, and legs.

Lie on your side on the floor or bed and place the ball on the side of your hip. Allow your body to relax onto the ball and let go of tension throughout your body so you end up draped over the ball. You may need to use some pillows to make sure you are comfortable (Figure 11.88).

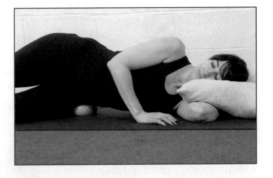

Figure 11.88: B8 – lying on the floor, place the ball under your hips. It should rest on the muscles at the top of your hip or any tender spots you find. Support yourself with a pillow for comfort.

As you lie on your hip you may feel pain and other sensations running up into your back or down into your leg. Explore other areas on the side of your hip to find the areas of restriction for you.

Myofascial ball work 9 (B9): Legs

You can use the balls anywhere on your legs, from the front of your hips to your calves, and on the sides as well.

The front of our hips is where our body hinges forwards. There are strong muscles and fascia deep in the hips which allow our body to hinge or flex forward. When we sit for long periods of time these become stuck and can pull our pelvis forward, creating an unnatural pressure on our lower back. The same muscles are also used when we walk, run, cycle, or pretty much do anything using our legs. There are also fascial connections from these muscles up into the diaphragm, which means that tightness in the front hips can affect your breathing.

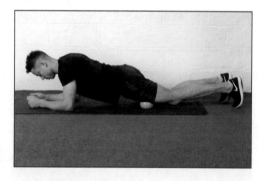

Figure 11.89: B9 – lying on your front on the floor, place one or two balls under the front of your thighs (so you can work on either one or both of your thighs together). Support yourself with your arms.

To release the front of your thighs, lie on the floor or bed and place the ball under your thigh. Allow your body to sink into the ball and slowly move to find the areas of tenderness and tightness. You can work anywhere from the top of your thigh where it attaches to the hip, down to just above your knee (Figures 11.89 and 11.90).

To release the back of your thighs, sit or lie on the floor or bed. If sitting have your legs out in front of you and your back supported (against a wall or sofa, or similar). Place the ball under your thigh and just allow the tissues to relax

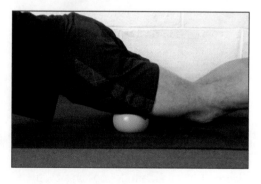

Figure 11.90: Close-up – allow time for your body to soften onto the ball(s).

and sink into the ball. Again, you can work anywhere from the top where the tissues attach into the pelvis right down to just above your knee (Figures 11.91–11.94).

To release your calves, sit on the floor or bed with your legs out in front of you and your back supported (against a wall or sofa, or similar). Place the ball under your calf and just allow the tissues to relax and sink into the ball. Again, you can work anywhere from just below to back of the knee down to your ankle (Figures 11.95 and 11.96).

To work on the sides of your legs, lie on your side and allow your body to rest on the ball. This area can be quite tender and you may not feel as much release here because the tissue is naturally thick and inelastic (Figures 11.97 and 11.98).

You can also work on the sides of your lower legs, again by lying on your side and allowing your leg to rest on the ball, working the ball into tender areas (Figures 11.99 and 11.100).

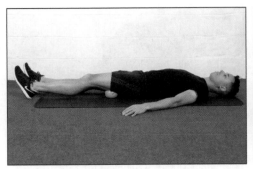

Figure 11.91: Lying on the floor, place either one or two balls under the back of your thighs.

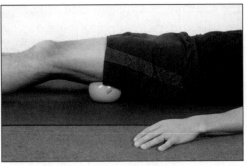

Figure 11.92: Close-up – allow time for your body to soften onto the ball(s).

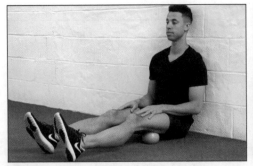

Figure 11.93: Alternatively you can sit with your back against a wall and either one or two balls under your thighs.

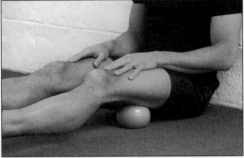

Figure 11.94: Close-up – allow time for your body to soften onto the ball(s).

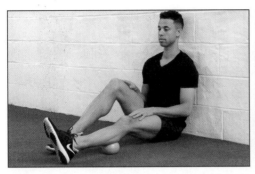

Figure 11.95: Sitting with your back against a wall or sofa, place either one or two balls under your calves.

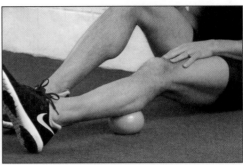

Figure 11.96: Close-up – allow time for your body to soften onto the ball(s).

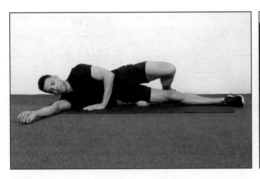

Figure 11.97: Lying on your side, place the ball under the side of your thigh. Support yourself with a pillow for comfort if necessary.

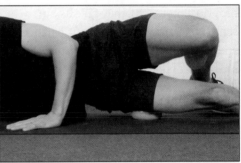

Figure 11.98: Close-up – allow time for your body to soften onto the ball.

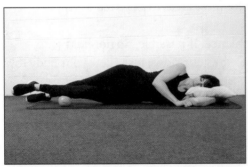

Figure 11.99: Lying on your side, place the ball under your shin. Support yourself with a pillow for comfort if necessary.

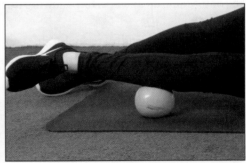

Figure 11.100: Close-up – allow time for your body to soften onto the ball.

Myofascial ball work 10 (B10): Feet

Our feet provide us with the stability to stand and to walk and run. They take the weight of our whole body. In many people their feet have become tight because of postural imbalances further up the chain in their body. Sometimes this causes dropped arches, where the fascia in the feet no longer supports the body correctly. The soles of the feet are also very sensitive, being full of proprioceptors, and they give us our sense of spatial awareness, our balance and our ability to move. Restrictions in the fascia of the soles of the feet can mean that we lose some of this proprioception and can become more clumsy, stumbling or losing our footing more easily.

To work on your bare feet, place the ball on the floor. While standing, roll the sole of your foot over the surface of the ball very slowly and mindfully. Pay attention to where things feel tender or restricted and pause on these areas until they release. You can roll onto your toes and heel too, allowing time for these areas to let go too.

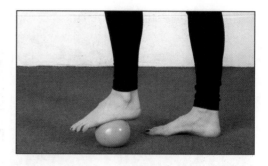

Figure 11.101: B10 – standing, place the ball under your bare foot. It is better to do this free standing, but if necessary hold onto something for support. Allow your arms to hang loose if possible.

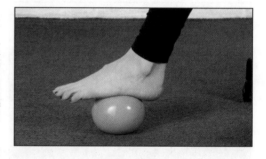

Figure 11.102: You can also work on your foot from a seated position. Again, allow your arms to hang loose.

As you work, be mindful to maintain your balance. If possible, do not hold onto anything and keep your arms hanging loosely by your sides; just allow your body to move and rebalance as the fascia releases.

Not only will this help to loosen the fascia in these areas, but you will find that you will start to feel a loosening all the way up your leg into your hip and even your back.

Using foam rollers

There has been much excitement in the sports and fitness world about using foam rollers for self-myofascial release. Many people who use them may be doing so without any therapeutic gain because they are almost certainly working too fast and too hard to do anything more than tenderize their muscles, in much the same way as a good steak hammer will do.

If you fancy having a go with a foam roller then first you get to choose your roller. Not all foam rollers are equal and there are two things to consider:

- hardness
- size.

Foam rollers vary in hardness and this is usually indicated by their color. Softer rollers, which are made of more porous foam, are usually green or blue, sometimes even pink or white. Harder rollers, made of denser foam, are usually black. Some rollers even come with added knobbly bits which makes them even harder.

You need a foam roller that suits your body. If you are a 95 kilo fit man, then a black foam roller will be strong enough to support your weight and give sufficient pressure. However, if you are a 55 kilo woman, or anyone with a lot of fascial restrictions, you will need a softer roller to give support but without causing you so much pain that you give up before you get through the first attempt.

Next let us talk about size. Foam rollers now come in all sorts of shapes and sizes. Standard lengths of roller vary from 30 cm to 90 cm. Shorter rollers are great for using on feet and harder to get to areas such as the underside of the arms and the inside legs. They are also more portable so you can take them to the office, for example. Longer rollers are good for bigger areas such as the back or legs, and you can also use them for whole body stretches (see the towel stretch above).

Most rollers are round so that actually rolling on them is easy. However, you can also get rollers in a half-moon shape. These are also good for lying on, and better for people with less mobility because they do not roll around as you get on and off them.

Having chosen your roller, this next thing to think about is speed. Just remember, fascial is slower – the slower the better. Remembering that fascia takes 90 to 120 seconds before it starts to release, you really want to be moving your body over your roller very slowly. As you do, you will discover areas that feel tighter and more painful. These are where you should stop and wait. Adjust the roller so that you are on the right spot, then adjust your weight and the rest of your body (using pillows or other supports as necessary), so you can maintain a steady gentle pressure, and wait for the tissues to release.

With practice you can use a foam roller in the same way you would use a myofascial ball. Therefore you can adapt any of the ball work exercises we recommend and do them with a foam roller. The technique is exactly the same and, so long as you are using the roller slowly and mindfully, you will achieve similar results. Although myofascial balls are great for smaller areas and rollers can really help with larger areas, often it is entirely a matter of personal preference whether you work with a ball or a roller.

Table 11.1 gives a summary of all the exercises in this chapter, listed by body area and typical conditions.

Table 11.1: Summary of all exercises by area and condition

Body area	Typical conditions	General activities	Fascial stretches	Myofascial ball work
Head and neck	Headaches, migraines, NDPH	Any	S1, S2, S3	B1, B2, B3
	Neck pain, torticollis, whiplash	Any	S1, S2, S3	B1, B2, B3
	Tinnitus	Any	S1, S2, S3	B1, B2, B3
	TMJ, jaw pain	Any	S1, S2, S3	B1, B2, B3
Neck, chest, and arms	RSI, thoracic outlet syndrome	Any	S1, S5, S6	B2, B4, B6
	RSI, golfer's elbow, tennis elbow	Any	S1, S4, S5	B2, B4, B5
	RSI, carpal tunnel syndrome, tendonitis	Any	S1, S2, S4	B2, B5, B6
	RSI, Dupuytren's contracture, trigger finger	Any	S1, S2, S4	B4, B5, B6
Shoulders	Rotator cuff injuries, frozen shoulder	Any	S1, S2, S6	B1, B3, B4
Back and pelvis	Upper, mid, or lower back pain, prolapsed and bulging discs	Any	S6, S7, S8	B3, B7, B8
	Sciatica, piriformis syndrome	Any	S7, S8, S10	B7, B8, B9
	Chronic pelvic pain syndrome, non-bacterial prostatitis	Any	S6, S7, S8	B7, B8, B9
	Chronic abdominal pain	Any	S6, S7, S8	B7, B8, B9
Legs and hips	Knee pain, runner's knee	Any	S8, S9, S10	B7, B8, B9
	Shin splints	Any	S8, S9, S10	B8, B9, B10
	Chronic compartment syndrome and calf pain	Any	S8, S9, S10	B8, B9, B10
	Plantar fasciitis, heel spurs	Any	S8, S9, S10	B8, B9, B10
Pain syndromes	Fibromyalgia, CFS, ME	G4, G5	S1, S2, S7	B1, B6, B10

NDPH, new daily persistent headache; RSI, repetitive strain injury; TMJ, temporomandibular joint; CFS, chronic fatigue syndrome; ME, myalgic encephalomyelitis.

Fascia in the Wider World

Health is a state of complete physical, mental and social well-being,
not merely the absence of disease or infirmity.

World Health Organization

This chapter includes suggestions on:

- how to create a more fascia-friendly workplace
- exercise you can do (discreetly) at work
- other fascia-friendly activities and movement therapies to try.

Once you become aware of your fascial health and start taking positive steps to improve it and help yourself out of chronic pain, it is likely that you may start to question the activities you do at work and in your leisure time. This chapter contains some suggestions to support you in the wider fascial world.

A more fascia-friendly workplace

We have already spoken at length about the restrictions of the modern workplace which in turn lead to the development of fascial restrictions.

Even if you do not have a desk job this will be relevant to you if you spend any time at a computer or laptop, at home on your tablet, or out and about with your phone.

The two main factors that cause fascial restrictions are:

- equipment
- movement.

Fascia-friendly equipment

Whether you work in an office, use a computer at home, or both, how much attention have you paid to the equipment you use? Not just your computer, but your desk, your chair, your lighting – all the other paraphernalia that is referred to as your workstation.

However much or little you use any kind of computing device, there is a wrong and a right way to go about it.

Many people who start a new office job inherit a desk, chair, screen, and keyboard from someone else. You may have been given a standard setup that everyone uses, or you may have a mixture of old and new equipment, things that work fine and things that maybe do not work so well. Most people sit down, switch on their computer and get started. But hold on a moment.

Everyone in the UK is legally entitled to a workstation assessment when they start a new job or any time they move location in their job. This includes people who work from home, people who hot desk, and people who work in production environments such as factories.

The purpose of the assessment is to ensure you have a safe place in which to work, but many people still develop fascial restrictions which lead to a chronic pain condition such as RSI. This is because:

- Often workstation assessments are just tick-box exercises designed so your employer can demonstrate they have complied with the basic law.
- Many of these assessments are based on assumptions and do not assess you as an individual, nor do they assess your changing needs.
- Unless you know the basic principles of correct equipment setup you cannot help yourself to stay fascially fit and healthy.

Keeping yourself fit and healthy at work requires a workstation that meets the following basic requirements:

1. Your chair. If you do nothing else, make sure you have a good chair. A correctly adjusted chair does not have arm rests, it allows you to get your body in under the desk, it supports your lumbar back, it supports your upper back, it has a seat pad that does not cut into the backs of your knees, and it moves as you move (in terms

of both the wheels and the actual chair components, swiveling so you do not have to twist, and adjusting forward and back as you shift your weight).

2. Adjust the rest of your workstation setup around your chair. For example, to have your elbows just above the desk and your shoulders relaxed (see below), you might find your feet dangling. If this is the case, use a foot rest rather than be tempted to drop the height of your chair.

3. Support your back. Many people think that you should not rest your back against the chair when working because sitting freely engages and strengthens your core muscles. This is fine if you are only working for a short period of time. But if you are in a job where most of your work is at a computer, your back and core will become fatigued pretty quickly without good support.

4. Relax while you work. Resting your arms on armrests or your desk while you type might feel comfortable but it is unhealthy for your fascia because it does not allow free movement of the whole of your arm. It also encourages overuse of the forearms, wrists, and hands, often in the incorrect position.

5. Your desk. In an ideal world your desk should be at the correct height to allow your chair to be correct too. There are many desks now that are adjustable to accommodate different people. There are even desks that can be converted to a standing desk as research shows that changing between two heights helps promote good posture.

6. You should be able to sit at your desk squarely, without being jammed in by desk drawer units, wastepaper bins or anything else that may inhibit your movement. And you should be able to access everything you need without having to twist repetitively (a sure-fire way to develop fascial restrictions in your lower back).

7. Easy access. Your screen, keyboard and mouse should all be within easy access. The screen should be setup so that the top of the screen is at your eye level or just below. Your keyboard should be directly in front of you, and your mouse at the side.

8. Your phone. If you use a phone a lot while working, get a headset. Cradling the phone between your ear and shoulder while you type will create fascial restrictions in your neck and shoulders and lead to RSI problems. If you work from documents regularly, get a document holder so that you can work without having to constantly look down or to one side.

9. Your environment. This may be less immediately obvious, but your work environment should have good lighting free from glare, and be at the right temperature and free from draughts. I have seen several clients with neck and shoulder pain caused by fascial restrictions formed as a result of sitting under an air conditioning vent.

10. Your eyes. If you wear glasses, make sure you have the correct prescription for reading a computer screen without straining your eyes. And did you know that in the UK you are entitled to a free eye test, even if you already wear glasses?

Adopting these principles will help you to stay healthy at your work, avoiding the build-up of fascial restrictions that can lead to chronic pain conditions. They are principles that you can adopt wherever and whenever you use a computer.

Fascia-friendly movement and exercises at work

Remembering that fascial fuzz starts to develop within 2 minutes of not moving (Chapter 6), you need to move your body regularly to break it down again. This does not mean that you need to break off from your work or interrupt meetings every couple of minutes to perform some intricate yoga poses. It is enough to introduce small movements simply to remind your body that it can move, as well as helping to keep your fascia healthy.

Try rolling your neck and shoulders to move the muscles and shift your fascial fuzz, or look away from your screen for a couple of minutes to let your eyes refocus (yes, you have fascia in your eyeballs). Stretching your arms is great.

Take any excuse to get up and walk about. Go and get yourself a glass of water (this helps to keep your fascia hydrated as well as moving), walk to the printer, get up to speak to a colleague instead of emailing them (warning: may not work if you are in London and they are in New York!). Go on, have fun finding discreet ways to stretch your fascia without anyone else knowing.

If you do not mind a bit of attention (and maybe one or two colleagues joining in), here are some great fascia-friendly movements you can do without fuss.

Neck rolls
Sitting at a computer screen for prolonged periods causes the fascia in your neck to tighten as it supports the weight of your immobile head. Neck rolls help to break up this tension.

Slowly rotate your head from side to side, keeping within a comfortable range of movement. Then start with your head to one side and tip your chin down to your chest and back up to the other side. Repeat in the other direction, but do not roll your head back as this can cause dizziness (Figures 12.1–12.3).

From an upright position, take your right ear to your right shoulder, then change and do the same on the left. Your shoulders should remain loose and relaxed so they

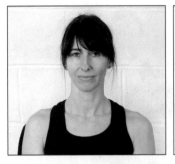

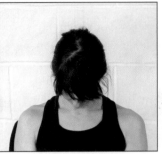

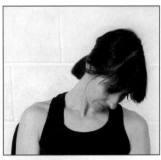

Figure 12.1: Neck roll – start position.

Figure 12.2: Neck roll – drop head towards chest.

Figure 12.3: Neck roll – roll head towards one shoulder and then the other.

are not joining in the movement. This one is perhaps best practiced in a mirror first to ensure your shoulders do not get in on the act (Figures 12.4 and 12.5).

Shoulder roll

Shoulders get tight as we sit using a computer. Without us realizing, our shoulders can end up hunched somewhere round our ears. Taking time to roll your shoulders out encourages them to return to a more relaxed position.

Either sitting or standing, keep your arms relaxed and roll both shoulders forwards and then backwards. (If it helps, imagine you are an old steam train powering your wheels forward in unison. You can make the noises too if you like (Figures 12.6–12.9)).

Arm and chest stretch

Sitting at a computer can cause our posture to collapse inwards, increasing tension in the fascia in our chest and causing desk-hunch.

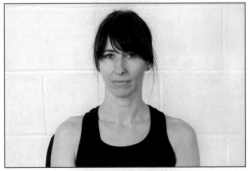

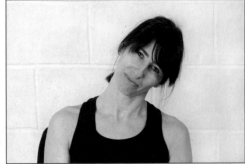

Figure 12.4: Neck stretch – start position.

Figure 12.5: Neck stretch – tilt head to one side and then the other.

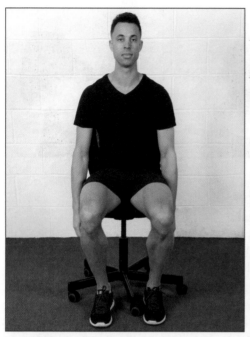

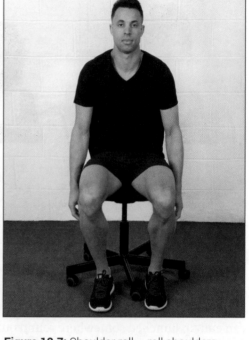

Figure 12.6: Shoulder roll – start position.

Figure 12.7: Shoulder roll – roll shoulders forward.

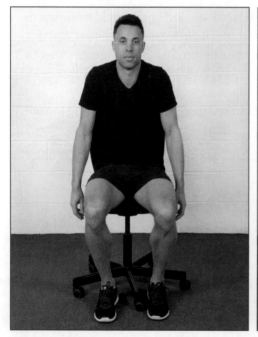

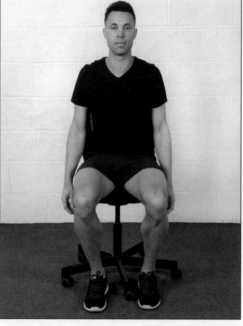

Figure 12.8: Shoulder roll – lift shoulders up to ears.

Figure 12.9: Shoulder roll – roll shoulders back and down to complete a circular movement.

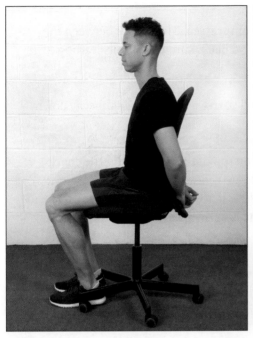 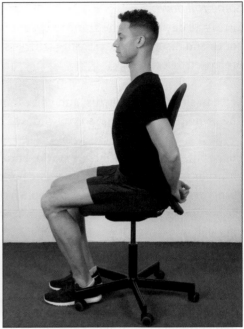

Figure 12.10: Arm and chest stretch – start position with hands clasped behind you and arms relaxed.

Figure 12.11: Arm and chest stretch – keeping hands clasped, stretch arms back and chest forward.

Either sitting or standing, take both arms behind your back (around your chair back if seated), interlace your fingers and stretch up, out and back. You should feel your back arching, your chest lifting and your shoulder blades coming together. This is a particularly good one to counteract contracted chest muscles from desk-hunch (Figures 12.10 and 12.11).

Arms and hands

Our arms and hands bear the brunt of our computer and mouse work. They spend too long stuck in one position so why not re-energize them with a bit of jiggling every now and then?

A great way to remind your arms that they can move is to shake them. Either sitting or standing, just let your arms and hands hang by your side and become as loose and floppy as you possibly can, and then shake them. Do it in whatever direction and at whatever speed you like. Shake it up a little to really loosen things up. It works from your fingertips to your shoulders and neck, and feels great too – very invigorating. Remember those jiggling atoms (Chapter 4)?

Spine roll down

Sitting all day causes the spine to become compressed. The spaces between the bones and discs reduce, creating stiffness and back pain, potentially leading to prolapsed discs.

You can sit or stand for this, and you can roll part-way down or all the way down. The principle is the same, so you choose.

Your spine is a series of bones stacked one on top of the other with little shock absorber pads between each one. The bones are called vertebrae and the shock absorbers are called discs. Most people have 24 vertebrae. The top one is just inside the bottom of your skull and the bottom one is at the base of your back just above your pelvis.

Each vertebra should move independently but in many people the vertebrae have become stuck together and can only move in groups. Over time this stuckness can lead to compressed bones and prolapsed discs (this is where a disc gets squeezed out from between its bones).

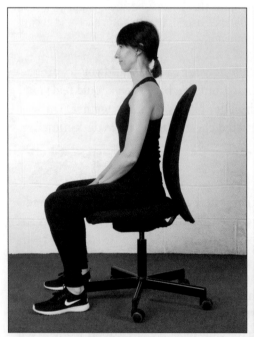

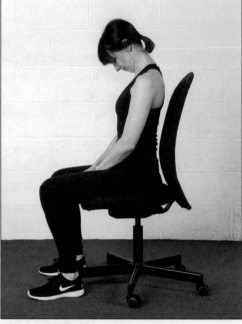

Figure 12.12: Seated spine roll-down start position – with your head level and legs spread to allow space for your body to roll down.

Figure 12.13: Seated roll-down – start by tipping your head forward and imagine your vertebrae rolling forward and down.

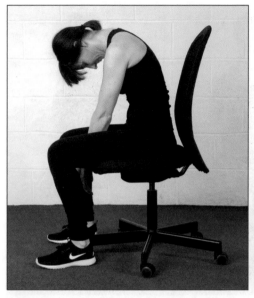 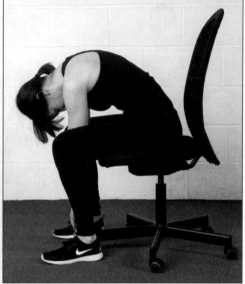

Figure 12.14: Seated part roll-down – finish position.

Figure 12.15: Seated full roll-down – finish position.

The idea with this exercise is to keep the bones moving independently one at a time. Starting at the top, breathe out slowly and as you do tip your head forwards, imagining each vertebra in the stack rolling forwards, one at a time. To ease the stretch, pause as you need to breathe in then keep rolling your vertebrae down as you breathe out. Keep yourself from slumping in the middle by breathing actively and deeply into your belly as you roll down. Just let your arms hang loosely throughout.

The trick with this exercise is to do it slowly and mindfully, because the more you do this, the more you will help your individual vertebrae to move independently.

If you are doing a part roll down, you will end up with your hands somewhere below your knees. If you are doing a full roll down, they will be somewhere near the floor. If you are doing this seated, you should spread your legs first to allow your body to roll right down.

Once you have rolled all the way down, wait there for a couple of slow deep breaths and then start to roll back up. This time, imagine each vertebra stacking back on top of the one below it, starting from your bottom vertebra and working up your back. Your head should be the last thing to come up and stack on the top.

Torso twist
This is another way to release your vertebrae and re-energize your body.

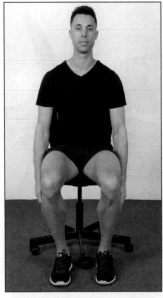
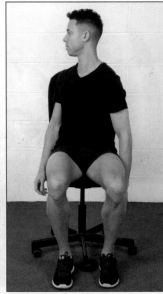
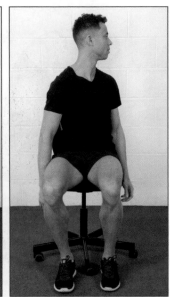

Figure 12.16: Seated torso twist – start position. Keep your arms loose.

Figure 12.17: Twisting to one side.

Figure 12.18: ...and then the other – if you do this with a bit of a swing, your fascia will warm up and loosen more.

Either seated or standing, twist your torso round to each side in turn. If you can, allow your arms to swing loosely as you twist, like a pair of pigtails by your side (Figures 12.16–12.18).

Pelvic tilt

Sitting twists the pelvis into an unnatural position, which can lead to lower back and leg pain. This helps to alleviate some of the strain.

Seated, focus on your pelvis. Sit upright, with your belly button pulled into towards your spine. Allow some space between you and the chair back to give your pelvis some room to move. This helps to isolate the movement of your pelvis without exaggerating the movement in other parts of your body.

Imagine your pelvic bones are a cradle and rock them forward. You may feel your back arch slightly, but stay as upright as possible. Then reverse the movement and tock your pelvic bones backward. You may feel your back round slightly as you do this, but again stay as upright as possible. This should feel like a rolling movement pivoting on your sitting bones (Figures 12.19–12.23).

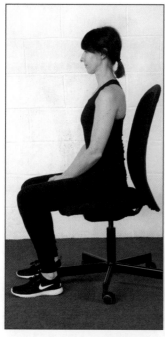 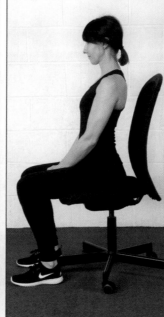 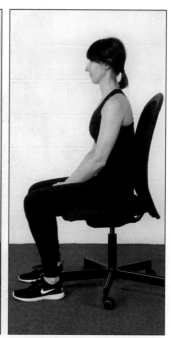

Figure 12.19: Seated pelvic tilt start position – sitting upright with your belly button pulled in towards your spine. Allow some space between you and the chair back to give your pelvis room to move.

Figure 12.20: Imagine your pelvic bones are a cradle and rock them forwards. You may feel your back arch slightly, but stay as upright as possible.

Figure 12.22: Now rock your pelvic bones backwards. You may feel your back round slightly as you do this, but stay as straight as possible.

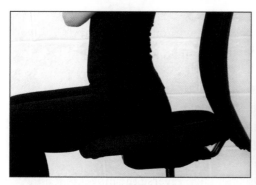 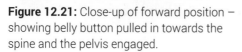 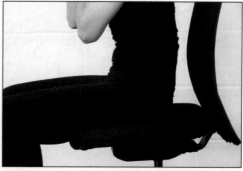

Figure 12.21: Close-up of forward position – showing belly button pulled in towards the spine and the pelvis engaged.

Figure 12.23: Close-up of backward position – showing belly button pulled in towards the spine and the pelvis engaged.

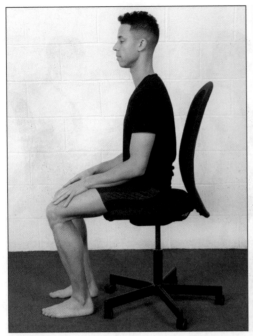 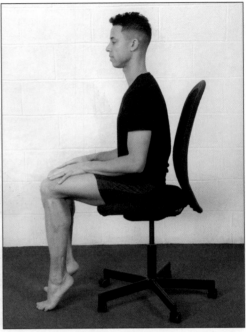

Figure 12.24: Seated calf raise start position with your feet flat on the floor. Take your shoes off to do this exercise for maximum benefit.

Figure 12.25: Lift your heels up bringing your feet onto your toes. Feel this in your calves. Drop your heels back down to the floor and repeat.

Calf raise

As well as being involved in walking, calves are responsible for pumping blood and other fluids back up from your legs to your heart. They can only do this when they are moving, so this exercise helps them do their job.

Seated, place your feet on the floor. This is best done without shoes on and definitely without heels – any shoes will inhibit movement of your feet and reduce the stretch.

Raise your heels up until you are on your toes and then allow them to gently come back down to the floor. Repeat a few times. This is a good one to get sluggish blood flowing again in the calves and lower leg (Figures 12.24 and 12.25).

Ankle rotation

As well as helping the calves (see previous exercise), this helps loosen the ankle joints.

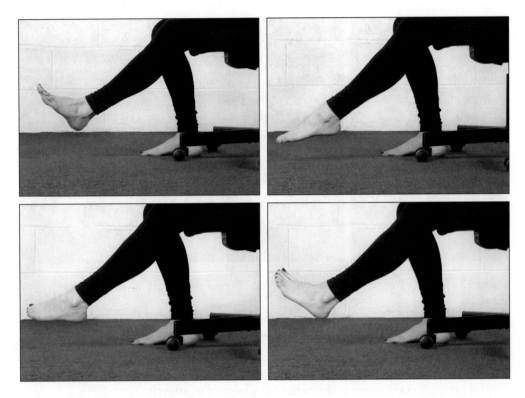

Figure 12.26: With your shoes off, take your ankles into a full circular rotation, rolling your foot clockwise and then anti-clockwise.

Seated, lift one foot off the floor and gently rotate your ankle in both directions – again this is best done without shoes on to allow full movement of your feet. Repeat for the other foot (Figure 12.26).

Foot twist

Feet get tired and tight when they are not moving. This exercise wakes them up and stretches the fascia from the foot to the knee.

Seated, and again without shoes, lift one foot off the floor and twist it so the sole of your foot faces inward and then outwards. Repeat for the other foot (Figure 12.27).

It is so easy to spend hours hunched over your tablet, slouching on the sofa or in bed, or at your desk without a break because you have a deadline. The reality is, however, the more you do this, the more likely you are to develop some kind of chronic pain condition because your body is simply not designed to behave in this way.

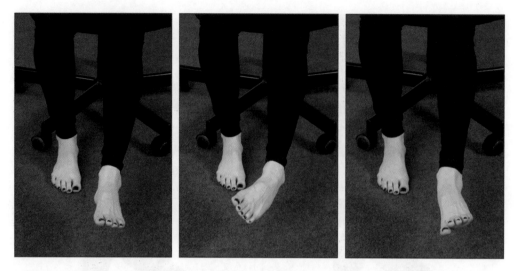

Figure 12.27: With your shoes off, twist your foot so the sole faces first inwards and then outwards.

However, if you become more mindful of what you are doing with your body at work and at play on any piece of computer equipment, you will start to notice the tightening in your fascia, the twinges, the aches that come and go, all of which are helpful reminders that your body wants to move and to stretch.

By stretching and moving regularly, you will counteract the stuckness in your body and remind your fascia that it can actually move freely.

Fascia-friendly cardiovascular exercise

In this chapter we have already touched on the effects of exercise on your fascia. In Chapter 6 we also looked at the injuries to fascia caused by both underuse and overuse. Modern lifestyles, with their many demands on our time, mean that it is difficult to get the balance right. Sensing their need to move, many people hit the gym or pound the pavement to counteract the effects of their immobile work day without considering the considerable impact this has on their fascial selves.

This 0 to 60 mph approach to exercise often means that fascia is ill-prepared for the demands put upon it and, rather than promoting health, instead it leads to injury.

This is not to say that we should not exercise. According to Public Health England, 43% of the UK adult population do no regular exercise at all, not even walking. This underuse is just as bad for our fascia. What is needed is a more considered and balanced approach to exercise.

Regular cardiovascular (CV) exercise is essential for good mental, physical, and therefore fascial health. From a physiological perspective, CV exercise provides the healthy stress that keeps our bodies working properly. It stimulates circulation, breathing, and muscle tone. It promotes the release of feel-good chemicals such as endorphins (see Chapter 7) which make us feel good and happy. And, once our exercise is over, this stimulates the rest and digest function, promoting good digestive health, tissue repair and sleep. Any exercise also means movement which keeps our fascia healthy and fluid.

CV exercise comes in many forms. It is something that you can gradually introduce into your daily routine. Remember, your fascia responds to gentle pressure (Chapter 11). Expect it run a marathon on day 1 and it will hit back. Bearing in mind the fact that it takes the body 6 months to replace your fascia, a gradual increase in the amount of regular CV exercise you do will ensure your fascia remains healthy and fluid.

Fascia-friendly CV exercise includes: walking, gentle jogging, swimming, cycling, gardening, and exercise classes. "Regular" CV exercise means doing whatever it is for at least 20 minutes three to five times a week. This means you get to choose what you fancy and mix it up a bit.

Walking to and from work, or even part of the way, is great fascia-friendly exercise and relaxation. If you choose this option then it is a good idea to invest in a good pair of trainers that support your feet and a good rucksack, rather than a bag slung over one shoulder (which is almost guaranteed to lead to postural imbalance). If walking to and from work is a step too far, what about taking the stairs when you get there, avoiding the queue for the lift, and flexing your fascia as you go.

Whatever CV exercise you decide to do, choose something that you actually like and that fits with your lifestyle so that it is not a chore and becomes part of your regular daily routine.

Other fascia-friendly activities and movement therapies to try

Fascia-friendly activities are those that help to move our fascia into balance and maintain it there. Fascia-friendly balance means using the natural tensegrity of your fascial body (Chapter 5), your fascia's natural ability to adjust and find its own healthy balance.

If your posture is incorrect, then you are not in balance. As we know (Chapter 6), poor posture and imbalance develop as a result of gradual, almost imperceptible tightening and restrictions in the fascia. These are caused by our body habits, our work, and our exercise. Over time each slight restriction creates a shift in the tensions conducted through our fascia, and gradually the body starts to tighten along the new lines of tension. These changes typically happen over years, gradually shifting a body into a posture that looks clearly imbalanced from the outside yet which feels perfectly normal to the person who has adjusted to it.

One of the most effective ways that you can help your mind, your body, and therefore your fascia to release and rebalance is through movement therapy. Therapies such as yoga, Pilates, Alexander technique, tai chi, and qi gung, to name a few.

Although these are all distinct forms of exercise, their practice and benefit is very similar. When practiced regularly, movement therapy works to promote improved posture and therefore balance. Through practice you will develop a deeper feel for your body position and your fascia, engage your core muscles to maintain balance, and cultivate a calmness and control of your breath that soothes your nervous system and keeps you moving.

Movement therapies also require a mental focus when practiced correctly – ask anyone who has been to a yoga class and tried to stand on one leg for any length of time. This mental focus literally takes your mind off things and helps to slow your thoughts, engaging your nervous system and easing you into rest and digest, when your body can carry out repairs.

Movement therapies have been around for centuries in many cases and they are the ultimate slow fix for wholistic mind–body health, having evolved through an understanding of fascia and that interconnectedness of every part of the mind–body.

I have lost count of the number of people I have seen who have combined their myofascial release therapy with an introduction to movement therapy. In virtually every case, they have expressed amazement at the power of their chosen therapy to release and rebalance their bodies. They also begin to notice how this contributes to a new mental calmness and sense of self-empowerment. These are often people who had previously thought that the only route to fitness was through endless weight training or punishing exercise routines. Once they discover movement therapy, they become calmer and develop a better appreciation of long-term health.

You get to choose the movement therapy that is right for you, so try a few classes and see what fits. I suggest you choose a small class size, maximum 10 people. Larger classes are fine for people who know what they are doing, but they are not good for a complete beginner, especially one who has chronic pain. It is a good idea to tell your teacher about your chronic pain and explain what movements you have difficulty with. For example, if you have RSI, some yoga poses may not be possible at first. A good teacher will always have alternatives for you to try.

Whatever combination of exercise and other activities you choose, regular and mindful practice will help to develop and maintain fascial balance in your body. Combined with the fascial activities, stretches and myofascial ball work exercises in this book, you have the choice now to create a healthy new fascial you.

Conclusion: Wrapping It All Up (in Fascia)

The doctor of the future will give no medicines but will interest his patients in the care of the human frame, in diet, and in the causes and prevention of disease.

Thomas Edison

A few final words of encouragement

As this book comes to an end, this is the start of your journey of fascial self-care and self-empowerment. Knowing what you now know about fascia, about the three-dimensional web that creates structure and communicates change in your mind–body, you can set out with confidence.

Knowledge really is power. By understanding how chronic pain develops and why it persists, you can make the changes that will break the chronic pain cycle. You have everything you need within you to release, rebalance, and re-create the space for your mind–body to heal itself.

As you start on your new fascial journey, remember that there may be setbacks, there may be days when you feel your pain is no better, but remember also that the key to working with fascia is the slow fix. It takes 6 months of regular self-care for your fascia to renew itself, so work slowly, work regularly, work mindfully and you will be rewarded with a new fascial you.

In this world where everything appears to be speeding up, where demands are becoming ever more urgent, you can be kind to yourself by allowing time to stretch, to breathe, and to move in a fascial way. By slowing down ever so slightly, maybe so slightly that only you are aware of it, you are giving yourself time to heal.

Thank you for joining me on my fascial journey. I wish you well on yours.

The future is fascia!

Some Suggested Further Reading

Barnes, J.F. 2000. *Healing Ancient Wounds: The Renegade's Wisdom.* MFR Treatment Centers, Malvern, PA.

Barral, J.P. & Mercier, P. 2005. *Visceral Manipulation, 2e.* Eastland Press, Vista, CA.

Becker, R.O. & Selden, G. 1998. *The Body Electric, 2e.* William Morrow, NY.

Chopra, D. & Pert, C. 1999. *Molecules of Emotion: Why You Feel the Way You Feel.* Simon & Schuster, NY.

Chopra, D. 2015. *Quantum Healing: Exploring the Frontiers of Mind/Body Medicine.* Bantam Books, NY.

Dispenza, J. 2014. *You are the Placebo: Making Your Mind Matter.* Hay House, London.

Levine, P. 1997. *Waking the Tiger: Healing Trauma – the Innate Capacity to Transform Overwhelming Experiences.* North Atlantic Books, Berkeley, CA.

Lipton, B.H. 2005. *The Biology of Belief: Unleashing the Power of Consciousness, Matter and Miracles.* Hay House, London.

Myers, T.W. 2013. *Anatomy Trains: Myofascial Meridians for Manual and Movement Therapists, 3e.* Elsevier, London.

Niel-Asher, S. 2014. *The Concise Book of Trigger Points, 3e.* Lotus Publishing, Chichester.

Oschman, J.L. 2000. *Energy Medicine: The Scientific Basis, 2e.* Churchill Livingstone, Edinburgh.

Pischinger, A. & Heine, H. 2007. *The Extracellular Matrix and Ground Regulation: Basis for a Holistic Biological Medicine.* North Atlantic Books, Berkeley, CA.

Pollack, G.H. 2001. *Cells, Gels and the Engines of Life: A New, Unifying Approach to Cell Function.* Ebner and Sons, Seattle, USA.

Schleip, R. & Baker, A. (eds.). 2015. *Fascia in Sport and Movement*. Handspring Publishing, Edinburgh.

Schleip, R. Findley, T. Chaitow, L. Huijing, P. (eds.). 2012. *The Tensional Network of the Human Body*, Elsevier, NY.

Stecco, L. 2004. *Fascial Manipulation for Musculoskeletal Pain*, Piccin, Italy.

Upledger, J.E. & Vredevoogd, J.D. 1983. *Craniosacral Therapy*, Eastland Press, Vista, CA.

Index

Myofascial Release Kit

Experience the great benefits of myofascial release for yourself with our easy to use kit

Contains 2 myofascial release balls,
1 soft bag, plus an information leaflet

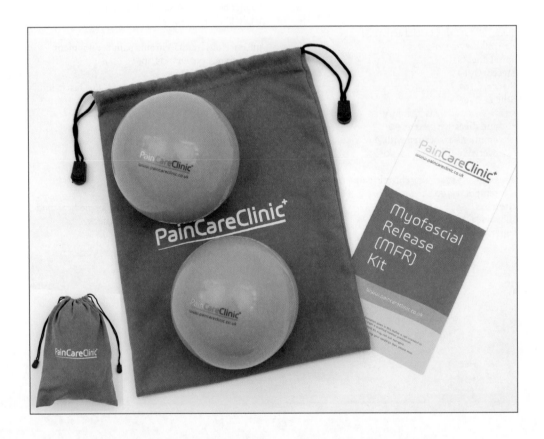

Available from paincareclinic.co.uk